The Awesome Foursome

The Essential Components of *Optimal Health & Total Fitness*

Irwin Schwartz, Ed.D., CSCS
with David H. Schwartz, Ph.D.

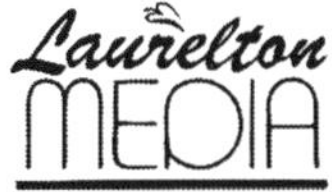

The Awesome Foursome
The Essential Components of Optimal Health & Total Fitness

Irwin Schwartz, Ed.D., CSCS
with David H. Schwartz, Ph.D.

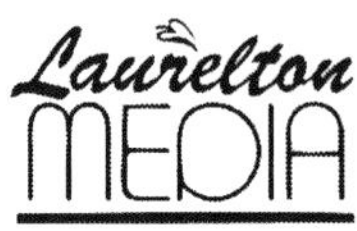

P.O. Box 660
Millwood, New York 10546
www.laureltonmedia.com
www.awesomefoursomebook.com

Editor: Natalie Schwartz
Copyeditor: Melissa Tammaro
Layout Editor: Laura Wurzel
Illustrator: Leo Sietz

Printed in the United States of America

Library of Congress Control Number: 2009911115
ISBN: 978-0-9816935-2-1

Dedication

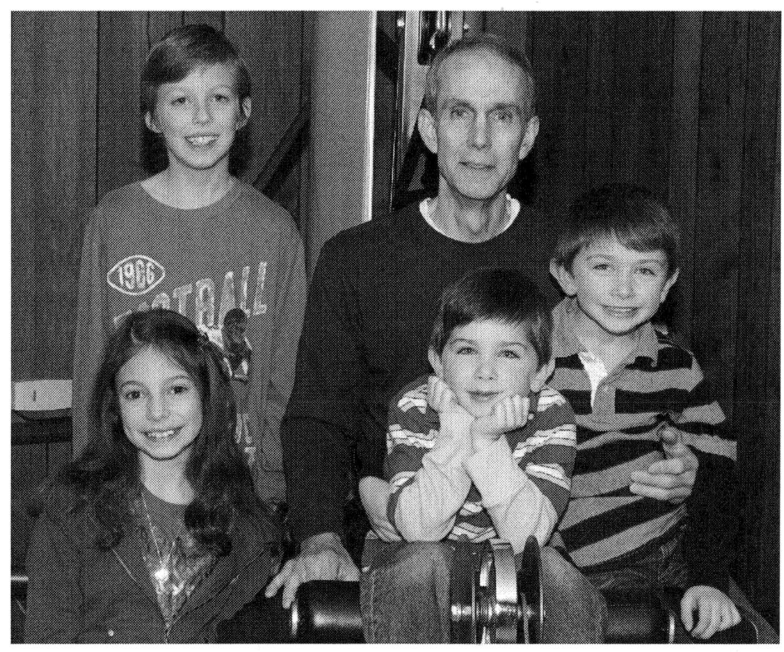

This book is dedicated to my
Awesome Foursome—my four grandchildren.

The Awesome Foursome

1. **Sensible Eating Lifestyle**
   A sensible eating lifestyle focuses on health, not weight.

2. **Cardiovascular Endurance Training**
   Regular aerobic exercise increases the efficiency of your cardiovascular system, enabling you to engage in physical activity for longer periods of time without becoming fatigued.

3. **Muscle Strength and Endurance Training**
   Weight training will not only improve your performance in sports and other physical activities, but it will also make your daily activities easier.

4. **Static Stretching for Flexibility**
   Engaging in static stretching will enhance your flexibility and help you avoid injury from physical activity as well as everyday movements.

Table of Contents

Preface

During my thirty-five years in the health and fitness industry, I've seen thousands of people stranded in a maze of health and fitness hype, pacing paths lined with miracles and magic potions. Their senses have been battered by an overabundance of information, advice and products that promise to deliver the ideal solution for achieving their health and fitness goals.

The simple yet comprehensive solution in this book cuts through the clutter. The unique message I convey to my students and clients stems from my educational background and professional experience as a health and fitness specialist, and from my personal experience practicing what I preach for the last three decades. This book encapsulates that message. I view it as a fitness seeker's guide out of the labyrinth and into the light of reason. In these pages you'll find a clear, practical roadmap for success that's based on research, generally accepted scientific findings, and my time-tested techniques.

When you embrace a total fitness lifestyle, you reap the rewards. Your ability to attain optimal health depends on your willingness to commit to a plan that fits your individual needs and circumstances. In this book you'll discover information that will enable you to make your exercise regimen efficient, safe and effective. You'll also find the motivation to embark on your journey toward total fitness.

Section I

Introduction

Chapter One

My Health and Fitness Philosophy

As children, all we did when we weren't in school was play. We played games our older siblings played, and we invented our own. We developed our own movement patterns, copied the way the older kids moved, and imitated the movements and gestures of our favorite athletes and entertainers.

As we got older, priorities changed and real life took over. For a number of reasons, many of us had to cut back on playtime. Eventually movement, once fluid and effortless, became forced and painful. The desire to play may have endured, but the body was unable to meet the physical demands of playing. For some, the decline was gradual and the only symptom was fatigue. But for others it was sudden, due to injury or illness, and the symptoms were pain and loss of movement.

We take medication for a broad range of ailments as a knee-jerk reaction, and we opt for cosmetic surgery in frightening numbers. When I read these statistics I'm reminded of a tee shirt I ordered from a magazine years ago. The following words were printed on the front: "Exercise is Medicine." I have worn that shirt to the first session of every one of my Wellness and Physical Fitness classes since 2000, and I will continue to wear it until one of us turns to dust. Perhaps we need to have a national advertising campaign to promote exercise as a modern miracle that makes you feel and look good, improves your health and fitness, and enables you to play like a kid again. Hey, it's noninvasive!

Some Introductory Thoughts

Health and *Fitness.* Are they the same, different? If you asked ten people, you'd get twelve different opinions.

To me, fitness is the state of being fit for something, fit for whatever you want to do. Too many people don't consider their level of fitness when they decide to play in the office softball game or in their town's tennis tournament. It doesn't occur to them that they haven't swung a bat or run around a tennis court for the last fifteen or twenty years. They forget or ignore that they've been sedentary for the twelve months or twelve years prior to the event. Emergency room physicians constantly hear things like, "I didn't think playing one time could cause this type of injury," or "I didn't even go all out."

The link between health and fitness is clear. When you are healthy, you have the potential to achieve the level of fitness required to participate safely in most of the physical activities that you enjoy.

Total fitness, as I define it, is the state achieved through healthful eating and an exercise regimen that includes aerobic exercise, weight training, and stretching for flexibility. It is a product of the interrelationships among these four variables, which I refer to as "The Awesome Foursome."

I have four criteria for adopting any workout or nutrition program: it must be physiologically sound, adaptable, effective and user-friendly.

Before you embark on your journey toward total fitness, you should assess where you are on the health and fitness continuum and where you would like to be. Positive movement along the continuum is sequential, progressive, and commensurate with effort. Though our goals may be similar, we all start at different points on the continuum and move at our own pace.

To exercise or not to exercise is, to a great extent, a question of priorities. But when considering where your health and fitness falls on your personal priority list, it can be helpful to think about the relationship between your health and your family's well-being. Don't wait for your doctor's stern-faced admonition.

Of course, going to the gym five, six or seven days a week and working out for two or three or more hours each day is not feasible for anyone but the most serious and dedicated individuals (e.g., competitive power lifters and bodybuilders). These dedicated athletes find or make the time to train.

This book is not for professional bodybuilders or power lifters. It was written for the millions of individuals who want to become fit for engaging in their favorite activities and improving their overall quality of life, but have not found a source that provides clear, concise guidelines and principles. This book is a roadmap dotted with comprehensive and detailed signposts and clear and concise informational markers that lead you on a successful journey toward optimal health and total fitness.

Speaking of Motivation

My wife and I raised three daughters. When our oldest got married, one of my three not-so-secret wishes—to become a grandfather—seemed destined to come true. My second wish—at least one grandson—was now a distinct possibility. Third, I wanted to continue playing baseball and to experience the joy of having my grandchildren come to my games.

In 1998 my first grandchild was born—a boy. Although I'd been adhering to a strict exercise regimen and sensible eating lifestyle since 1982, his birth was a powerful incentive to continue taking care of my health and staying fit as I got older.

I now have three grandsons and one granddaughter. It's hard for me to believe, but my eleven-year-old grandson has been coming to my games and sitting in the dugout with the team for the last five years. As much as he enjoys it, I suspect his presence means more to me than it does to him. I coach his baseball and basketball teams, and watch my six-year-old grandson play baseball and soccer. My granddaughter is also athletic, and I would be thrilled to see her budding interest blossom into an active motivation to participate in sports. They are now my most important team, and I will do everything in my power to see every inning of every game they play.

I'm proud to say that the 2009 baseball season marked my fifty-first consecutive season playing organized baseball or fast pitch softball. I pitch for the Astros in what was, until the 2008 season, the 28+ division of the

Westchester/Putnam Men's Senior Baseball League. As of 2008, the league has two divisions: 25 to 34 and 35+.

Because it gets a bit more difficult each year to keep up with the youngsters, and because they seem to keep getting younger, I've had to increase the intensity of my workouts. But it's well worth the effort. As we used to say in the Bronx: "If you keep on keepin' on, you can keep on keepin' on." I feel like I'm living proof.

Maintaining my good health and high level of fitness enables me to engage in the activities I enjoy, such as playing baseball, playing with my grandchildren, coaching youth sports, and occasionally playing a game of basketball without worrying that I can't keep up. Your motivations may be different from mine. Maybe you want to finish a marathon, cycle across the French Pyrenees, or simply improve the quality of your life. But with desire, drive, and the guidance this book provides, your level of success is limited only by your will and commitment.

The Excuses

You can always find an excuse: "I'm too old to change the shape of my body, and even if I could, it would never look like that." Although the latter part of that statement may be true, a sensible eating lifestyle and exercise will improve both the quality and longevity of your life.

Here are some other excuses: "I can't change the shape of my body, get stronger, or become more flexible because of my old injury," "because of my weight," or "because of a medical condition." There's almost always a way to achieve your goals. If you are unable to do one exercise, you can choose another option. Adaptation is the key. These excuses simply highlight the importance of speaking with your physician and seeking out trainers with the knowledge and experience to help you get started and progress. As for the weight issue, a sensible eating lifestyle, in combination with aerobic exercise, weight training, and stretching for flexibility, is the only viable answer. If you want to lose weight and keep it off, the principles in this book offer the safest, healthiest way to realize that goal.

Another favorite excuse: "Where am I going to find the time?" How badly do you want it? We need to prioritize with the big picture in mind. A healthy lifestyle requires a healthy balance among all of the things that compete for your time.

I have personally faced the obstacles and time constraints that sometimes turn the goal of getting healthy and fit into a real pain in the glutes. But whenever I'm confronted with an impediment, I remind myself that achieving this goal goes far beyond my appearance or my ability to throw a curveball. It impacts every facet of my life, from how I feel to how I think about the past, the present, and the future.

Overcoming the Inertia

Regardless of your situation and your goals, finding the time to exercise and eat sensibly is certainly a challenge. The highest hurdle can be getting started. It's a daunting task.

In your quest for health and fitness you face a multitude of obstacles and foes that are multi-faceted and unrelenting. Many of them we cannot see or touch, and yet we can certainly feel their impact. Examples include pathogens, air pollution, the stresses of everyday life, ads and commercials for fast foods, promos and infomercials (hyping everything from clothing to fitness products), procrastination, preconceived notions, and mismanaged priorities.

This book is designed to help you get past those obstacles and actually get started and continue in a sequential and progressive manner. It provides you with the information and education you need to attain total fitness.

Anyone who tells you getting and staying fit is easy has probably never tried it. Not only is it hard work to do the exercises, it's often harder to find the time. The most difficult part, however, is making the decision to do it. Once you make the decision, you'll be surprised at how much time you suddenly have available.

The Tale of the Scale

Most people focus on restricting their caloric intake when they want to lose weight. This approach is a mistake for two reasons. First, it doesn't take into account the types and sources of calories your body needs to be healthy. Only a sensible eating lifestyle, not a diet, will ensure your body is properly nourished and has the energy it needs to engage in physical activity.

The second problem with focusing on caloric intake to manage weight is it neglects the importance of regular exercise. Losing and gaining weight is a 50-50 proposition between the calories that come into the body in the form of food and the calories that the body burns when engaging in physical activity. Thus the best way to control your weight is to adopt a sensible eating lifestyle and engage in regular exercise.

You should also be aware that losing weight will not automatically enhance your health. It will not improve the shape of your body, make you stronger or more flexible, or strengthen your heart. Changing the composition of your body (i.e., the ratio of excess fat to lean body mass/muscle) will do all these things. Muscle weighs more than fat but takes up less room. Thus, if you raise the percentage of lean body mass and lower the percentage of excess fat, you might gain a couple of pounds, but you will lose inches and certainly look and feel better. You might even have to invest in a new wardrobe.

Basically, the most effective way to lose weight is to engage in all four components of The Awesome Foursome—a sensible eating lifestyle, cardiovascular endurance training, muscle strength and endurance training, and static stretching for flexibility. In fact, The Awesome Foursome will improve your overall health and fitness.

Chapter Two

The Awesome Foursome

Optimal health and total fitness have four key components, which I call The Awesome Foursome: (1) a sensible eating lifestyle, (2) cardiovascular endurance training, (3) muscle strength and endurance training, (4) static stretching for flexibility. Sections two through five of this book are each devoted to discussing one of these. Following is a basic overview.

Sensible Eating Lifestyle

Food is the fuel used by our bodies. The nutrients in food provide us with everything from a healthy immune system to strong bones and teeth to the energy required to work, play and think. Yet many people are on a quest to limit the food they eat. And so they diet. However, diets are inherently unhealthy, potentially dangerous, and, perhaps surprisingly, a major cause of obesity. With the exception of medically supervised diets, there is little to no scientific basis for the long-term success of diets. In most cases, diets are doomed to fail from the start. Most diets involve taking in too much of one type of nutrient and not enough (or none) of other essential nutrients. The simple fact that you cannot remain on a diet forever should raise a red flag.

Thus, instead of referring to the eating guidelines I describe in this book as a "diet," I refer to them as a "sensible eating lifestyle." Adopting a sensible eating lifestyle will ensure that you are getting all of the nutrition that you need, while allowing penalty-free cheating. Built into any sensible eating lifestyle are "discretionary calories" (e.g., desserts). In Section II: Sensible Eating Lifestyle, I provide you with a basic education on nutritional science and offer some simple and easy guidelines that you can follow for the rest of your life.

Cardiovascular Endurance Training

Wouldn't it be great if you could get to the top of a long flight of stairs without having to cling to the rail, gasping for air? The heart is the muscle responsible for pumping blood to all the other muscles and organs in the body. You strengthen your heart, which is cardiac muscle, by doing aerobic exercise. When you do aerobic exercise with the proper intensity, duration and frequency, you increase cardiovascular endurance and develop the stamina to do the things you want to do. In Section III: Cardiovascular Endurance Training, I discuss the basic physiology of the cardiovascular system, describe important principles, such as getting into your "target zone," and explain how to apply them to your training.

Muscle Strength and Endurance Training

Bones move, but it is the contractions of muscles that power that movement. Through weight training, you can develop two muscle characteristics: strength and local muscular endurance. In Section IV: Muscle Strength and Endurance Training, I describe how weight training can increase strength and local muscular endurance, and discuss the effect of nutrition and exercise on two other muscle characteristics: tone and definition. The section includes pictures of each of the basic exercises, along with comprehensive written descriptions. I combine these exercises to create different workouts targeted toward specific goals.

Static Stretching for Flexibility

Static stretching is done after a workout, when muscles are warm, to increase the range of motion around joints, and to serve as a cool-down. In Section V: Static Stretching for Flexibility, I provide you with pictures and detailed descriptions of how to do the stretches I consider necessary for all-around flexibility. I also explain why it's critical to adhere to proper form when stretching.

The Awesome Foursome: Working Together

Incorporating all four components of The Awesome Foursome into your lifestyle is the most effective way to achieve total fitness. This is because each individual component enhances the effectiveness of the other three. Let me explain:

A more efficient cardiovascular system positively influences both muscle strength and endurance, and flexibility. A strong heart can deliver more oxygenated blood with each beat, which decreases the number of beats per minute. Therefore, the heart has more available rest time between beats. More oxygenated blood enables muscles to work harder for longer periods of time without fatiguing. Increased blood flow brings warmth to the muscles, making them more supple. It also helps with the removal of waste products, which may decrease muscle soreness. These factors make static stretching easier and more effective, which improves flexibility.

Similarly, increased muscle strength and endurance benefits both the quality and quantity of aerobic exercise. Stronger leg muscles that won't tire quickly (local muscular endurance) will enable you to perform aerobic activities for longer periods of time and at higher intensity levels as you progress.

Increased flexibility is critical for the development of the other two exercise components of The Awesome Foursome: cardiovascular endurance and muscle strength and endurance. Since stretching increases the range of motion around joints, elongated muscles can be toned and strengthened along their entire lengths with a significantly decreased potential for injury. In addition, increased flexibility will improve your ability to perform your cardiovascular endurance workout effectively and efficiently. Stretching also serves as a cool-down after your cardiovascular and muscle strength and endurance training, an important bonus.

Finally, a sensible eating lifestyle will enhance your performance of the three exercise components of The Awesome Foursome. Nutrients in food provide the sustained energy necessary to lift weights, perform aerobic exercise, stretch, or engage in any type of physical activity. Proper nutrition is particularly relevant to weight training. Nutrients aid in the repair of body tissue (i.e., the microscopic tears in muscle fibers caused by weight training). The cumulative effect of these repairs, over time, is stronger muscles that will not tire quickly.

Some people who are dieting also exercise, but it's usually aerobic exercise they choose to do. While they are certainly on the right track, adding weight training will burn a lot of extra calories twenty-four hours a day by speeding up your metabolism. This is because muscles require fuel (in the form of calories) to contract and maintain tone. When you want to lose weight, it is most effective to engage in all four components of The Awesome Foursome.

Basically, excluding any one of the four components of The Awesome Foursome will severely diminish the benefits of the other three. It would be like arbitrarily deciding to change your car's oil but not the filter. You have to do both to reap the benefits of a well running car. To achieve optimal health and total fitness, you have to engage in all four components of The Awesome Foursome.

Chapter Three

Guide to Using This Book

The four sections that follow address the essential components of optimal health and total fitness. The order in which each component of The Awesome Foursome appears in this book is intentional and important. A sensible eating lifestyle (Section II) is the foundation of any fitness program; therefore, it is presented first. Cardiovascular endurance training (Section III) is discussed next because you need to engage in some form of aerobic exercise to warm up your muscles before you move on to muscle strength and endurance training (Section IV). Static stretching for flexibility (Section V) is presented last because it serves as a cool-down at the end of your total fitness workout.

I encourage you to read each section from the beginning to the end (as opposed to skipping around within a section). In each section, I provide a sequential progression of the key principles and concepts pertinent to that section.

You will also find illustrations of the proper way to do each of the weight training exercises and stretches. I encourage you to bring this book to the gym with you to use as a reference guide.

Please visit the website awesomefoursomebook.com for more information and to download useful reference guides and worksheets.

Now you know my health and fitness philosophy, you have an understanding of The Awesome Foursome, and you have a sense of how you can use this book. All that's left is to turn the page and get moving.

Section II

Sensible Eating Lifestyle

Chapter Four

A New Food Attitude

Developing eating habits that are consistent with sound scientific and medical principles is essential for achieving optimal health. Many people turn to fad diets and other nutritionally restrictive dietary programs in an effort to lose weight and improve their overall health. But these programs result in eating habits that are unhealthy.

My approach is to adopt a "sensible eating lifestyle." A sensible eating lifestyle focuses on health, not weight. Unlike a diet, a sensible eating lifestyle is a regimen you can follow for a lifetime. And it's easy. You don't need to count calories, measure portions or weigh food. Another plus: you can enjoy guilt-free indulgences, such as your favorite rich dessert or salty snack. This doesn't mean you can binge on sweets and fried foods. But when you follow the guidelines that I provide in Chapter Five, you'll see there is room for such calories.

Before we get to the guidelines, you have to change your mindset when it comes to what and how much you eat. In this chapter, I'll explain how to make fundamental changes in the way you relate to eating. To follow a sensible eating lifestyle, you must adjust your attitude toward food and eating by doing the following:

- Maximize your awareness of what you eat.
- Focus on the types of calories you consume (instead of the total number of calories).
- Forget diets.
- Change your preconceptions about meals.

Maximize Your Awareness of What You Eat

A recent scientific study found that participants lost weight when they maintained a food diary ("Keeping a Food Diary Doubles Weight Loss Results," Tufts University Heath & Nutrition Letter, October 2008). Every semester in my Wellness and Physical Fitness class I do an abbreviated version of this study. I ask my students to keep a log of everything they eat and drink over the course of three days. The students are usually astonished by what they find. It turns out that they never realized what they were eating or how much. They were never required to recall or review what they ate before. Some students find they take in a high number of calories from unhealthy sources, such as fast foods. Others realize they're taking in too few calories. But these two groups typically share one trait: they frequently feel run down and suffer from common ailments, such as colds. Once they become aware of their unhealthy eating patterns and the link to how they feel, they are more likely to change them.

Many diets require you to weigh your food or count calories. I don't advocate either of these approaches. Awareness and common sense, rather than convoluted and time consuming mathematical calculations, should be your guide. You don't need to keep a food diary either. Just be aware of what you're cooking or ordering at meal times and what you're grabbing at snack times. If you're mindful of what you're about to eat and the potential effect on your health, you're likely to make better choices. (To maximize your awareness of what you eat, use the food diary in Appendix One.)

Focus on the Types of Calories You Consume

A calorie is a unit of measurement for the energy released when the body breaks down the chemical bonds of food. Your tendency to gain or lose weight is driven by the relationship between the number of calories you take in and the number of calories you expend. But the source of calories is also an important part of the equation. Your body needs carbohydrates, proteins and fats to function properly.

Carbohydrates are sugars (simple carbohydrates) or starches (complex carbohydrates). They're found in potatoes, whole grains, fruits, vegetables, rice, pasta and table sugar. Fat is found in foods coming from animals, as well as from oils and butter. Protein is found in nuts, lean animal tissue, fish and beans.

Certain types of carbohydrates, proteins and fats are better for you than others, as you'll see in the following discussion.

Carbohydrates

Carbohydrates are the most readily available source of fuel because they're stored as glucose in the muscles where they're needed. Carbohydrates are used by the body for activities that require strength, power and endurance. Protein is also a source of energy, but it is used by the body only when carbohydrates and fats (discussed later) are not available. For example, the body may begin to break down its own muscle for protein when engaged in high intensity, long-duration activities. This can cause the degradation and loss of muscle tissue, leading to severe medical problems. Thus, you want to make sure you consume enough complex carbohydrates (and fats) to avoid exhausting your supply of stored energy. Carbohydrates are the nutritional foundation of your sensible eating lifestyle and your quickest supplier of fuel.

Foods rich in carbohydrates should make up the bulk of your diet. But not all carbohydrates are created equal. Complex carbohydrates, such as whole grain breads, cereals and pasta (i.e., foods that come from wheat, oats and rye) are healthful because they contain other nutrients, such as vitamins and minerals. They're also rich in fiber. When grains go through the refining process, the bran, which contains an abundance of fiber, is removed. That's why refined bread and pasta are not as healthful as the whole wheat options. Diets high in fiber can lower blood pressure, reduce susceptibility to digestive problems, and diminish the risk of heart disease and diabetes. Another plus: foods high in fiber fill you up and reduce the urge to snack and overeat.

Vegetables are also excellent sources of complex carbohydrates. Almost all fruits contain fructose, which technically is a simple sugar. But because the amount of simple sugar contained in most fruits is relatively low, fruits are good sources of carbohydrates. Also, most fruits contain other nutrients that are healthy (e.g., vitamins, minerals and antioxidants), and they're rich in fiber and low in fat.

Foods that contain simple sugars, such as white bread, white pasta and sugary snacks, are simple carbohydrates. They have more calories and a lower content of protein, vitamins, minerals and fiber compared to whole grain products. The body can break down simple sugars to provide energy, but for only a short period of time.

Fats

Foods that are high in fat are satisfying—they taste good and fill us up. Some are even known as comfort foods. But fats have a bad reputation because they're associated with gaining weight.

However, like carbohydrates, fats come in healthful and non-healthful options. Unsaturated fats have health benefits. They lower your LDL cholesterol level (LDL is known as the "bad" cholesterol, while HDL is the "good" one). Unsaturated fats can be divided into two broad categories: (1) monounsaturated fats, which are found in such oils as olive, peanut and canola; (2) polyunsaturated fats, which are found in such oils as corn, safflower and walnut.

Saturated fats, meanwhile, raise LDL cholesterol and have been linked to heart disease. Examples include meat and dairy products, such as cheese and butter.

The process of hydrogenation changes unsaturated fats into trans fats. Trans fats (trans fatty acids) not only raise the level of LDL but also lower the level of HDL in your body, increasing your risk of coronary heart disease (CHD). Many foods today contain partially hydrogenated oils and shortenings including cakes, cookies, crackers, potato chips, french fries and doughnuts.

Proteins

Protein is the structural core of the human body, and a protein deficiency can cause medical problems. However, it's easy to get the minimal daily requirement of protein in the United States and other developed countries. In fact, I don't recommend you take protein supplements or actively seek out additional sources of protein. Diets that call for drastically increasing protein consumption can cause potentially serious medical problems for two reasons: (1) High protein diets tend to be high in saturated fats and low in complex carbohydrates; (2) High protein diets can overwhelm the kidneys, which are responsible for filtering out protein.

Proteins can be found in meat, fish, poultry, eggs, dairy products including milk, and most beans and nuts. Animal sources of protein are also high in saturated fats, so it's a good idea to reduce your consumption of meats to lower your fat intake.

For more information on carbohydrates, fats, proteins, and other food groups, consult the United States Department of Agriculture's website at MyPyramid.gov. The website offers the latest dietary guidelines from the Center for Nutrition Policy and Promotion.

Forget Diets

Diets have been around for centuries. In an effort to lose weight, William the Conqueror, in 1087, locked himself in his room, ate nothing, and drank only alcohol. Hundreds of years later, an art dealer in 1903 advocated chewing each mouthful of food thirty-two times (once for each tooth), then spitting it out. He claimed you could get the nutritive value of food, and taste its flavor, without swallowing it.

Over the last two decades, low carbohydrate diets have become a major trend. These diets require you to drastically reduce your intake of carbohydrates and replace them with foods containing protein and fat. As I noted earlier, carbohydrates are an important source of fuel for the body. Thus, restricting carbohydrates is not a good idea.

You can't attain your long-term goal of optimal health and total fitness through dieting. It's unlikely you'll maintain your weight following the diet, and you may develop health problems. You can't stay on any diet indefinitely, which should send up a red flag. The sensible eating lifestyle I advocate is a long-term plan that allows you to remain healthy and fit for a lifetime.

Yo-Yo Dieting Won't Keep Off Pounds

Although diets are generally ineffective, unhealthy and potentially harmful, the dieting craze continues. In fact, the average woman goes on more than one hundred diets for five weeks on average, amounting to nearly ten years of her life, according to the Tufts University Health and Nutrition Letter ("Did You Know," Tufts University Health & Nutrition Letter, April 2009.)

Chronic dieting, or cycling on and off diets, is a phenomenon known as yo-yo dieting. Yo-yo dieting fails to keep weight off and can even lead to additional weight gain in the long run.

Diets Can Be Detrimental to Your Health

The potential risks associated with dieting far exceed their supposed benefits. As noted earlier, the most popular diets require that you take in mostly fat, saturated fat and protein, but little or no carbohydrates. These low-carb diets are dangerous because they cause potentially unfavorable changes in LDL cholesterol levels. They may also lead to health conditions associated with elevated ketosis—a crisis response of the body when it faces low dietary carbohydrate intake.

Low-carb diets may also impact your mental health because they deprive the brain of a necessary nutrient—glucose. Glucose is produced when the body breaks down carbohydrates. The glucose is then stored in your muscles so that it is immediately available for energy when needed. Glucose is also the brain's primary fuel. But the brain doesn't store glucose; it must be constantly available for optimal brain function.

Meanwhile, low-fat diet strategies may be contributing to the obesity epidemic in America because they require the dieter to focus on avoiding fat rather than managing their total caloric intake. In addition, these diets don't distinguish between unsaturated fats, which have health benefits, and saturated fats.

Change Your Preconceptions About Meals

A sensible eating lifestyle is all about consuming an adequate number of calories from a variety of nutritious sources. The custom of eating breakfast, lunch and dinner may work for you. But you can also consider a less rigid approach. Eating four to six times a day may fit your schedule better. Just make sure you fulfill your body's nutritional requirements by the end of the day.

One of the benefits of the traditional three-meals-a-day approach is that it keeps you on a regular schedule. If you're going to break with tradition, make sure you don't go more than four hours without eating. If you know you have a busy schedule on a particular day, be sure to pack portable, nutritious snacks.

You can always fill the nutrient gap with a mini meal at the end of the day. One of the most convenient times to eat is before going to sleep, although you should allow enough time to pass so that you will be comfortable lying down. The notion of eating before bedtime has often been associated with causing weight gain and other negative health effects. But I don't know of any scientific study demonstrating that it's any better or worse, from a nutritional or health standpoint, to eat before you go to sleep, compared to any other time of the day or night. If you're consuming extra calories before going to bed, it may lead to weight gain, but not because you consumed them at bedtime.

About Snacks and Desserts

Most people think of a snack as a tasty treat you eat between meals, and a dessert as a tasty treat you eat directly after a meal. In general, both are considered fattening and unhealthy. If you're going to change your perception of meals, you're going to need to change your perception of snacks and desserts as well.

Desserts and snacks don't have to be fattening and unhealthy. Instead of high-fat, sugary snacks, why not try snacking on a bowl of whole grain cereal with fresh fruit or low-fat yogurt with granola. Instead of fruit cocktail in heavy syrup, stick to fresh fruit. Instead of creamy dips, dunk veggies—such as broccoli, cauliflower, carrot sticks, green peppers, and red peppers—into low-fat yogurt.

But even high-fat, sugary desserts and salty snacks have a place in your sensible eating lifestyle. As long as you're satisfying all of your nutritional requirements for the day, the occasional indulgence is okay.

Keep in mind, you don't want to overindulge in sweets and other junk food because this can lead to weight gain and health problems. But if most of your calories are coming from complex carbohydrates, fruits and vegetables (which provide fiber), you're not likely to overindulge because these foods fill you up and satiate your hunger.

You can also prevent overindulging by eating only when you're hungry. Avoid eating when you're bored, to relax, to reduce feelings of anxiety, or to relieve stress

Always Eat Something Before You Start Your Day

You've heard it many times: "Breakfast is the most important meal of the day." Yet many people go well into the day before eating anything. I often hear things like "I'm in meetings all day" or "I have classes all morning."

Even if you're changing your approach to meal times and eliminating the traditional notion of breakfast, lunch and dinner, it's still critical to eat something before you start your day. You've just slept for hours, and your body may not have enough stored energy left from the previous day. It's like trying to start your car with an empty gas tank. You may go further than your car, but you'll soon feel wiped out.

In addition to providing you with the energy needed to start your day and function optimally, a wholesome breakfast helps you resist overeating later in the day. According to one study, the more calories you consume at breakfast, the less total number of calories you consume by the end of the day ("For Your Weight Control Effort, Breakfast - Eating More in the Morning May Help Limit Overeating at Night," Tufts University Health & Nutrition Letter, March 2004). Studies have also shown that individuals who eat a healthy breakfast are more likely to have a healthier diet overall and are less likely to be overweight.

Chapter Five

Sensible Eating Made Easy

Now that you understand why proper nutrition is important and how you should change your approach to eating, let's discuss the guidelines for maintaining a sensible eating lifestyle. While my guidelines are based on scientific research, I don't recommend you weigh food, measure portions, or scrutinize food labels, as other guidelines and nutritional programs do, because it's just not practical or time efficient. My guidelines are based on what the medical community knows about nutrition, but are flexible, easy to remember, and simple to follow:

- Increase your intake of whole grain foods.
- Reduce your consumption of simple sugars and sodium (salt).
- Substitute monounsaturated and polyunsaturated fats for saturated fats.

◆ Eat more fruits and vegetables.

You'll notice these guidelines involve making choices. If you're aware of what you're about to eat, as suggested in the previous chapter, you may find yourself making better choices.

Increase Your Intake of Whole Grain Foods

Most people don't consume enough complex carbohydrates. Many of my students complain that they feel run down, get colds frequently, or just don't feel as good as they'd like to. These are college students, young adults who should have plenty of energy. In fact, many of them are athletes.

As noted earlier, I ask them to record everything they eat and drink for three days. After reviewing their diet logs, I'm not surprised to discover the percentage of calories they consume from carbohydrates is too low, and the percentage of calories they derive from fat, saturated fat and protein is too high. The solution is not to eat more carbohydrates. The solution is to eat more complex carbohydrates in the form of whole grains.

Complex carbohydrates provide stored energy that's quickly accessible, fueling an active lifestyle. An added benefit: they're filling, curbing the urge to indulge in fast foods and sweet desserts.

Not all of your carbohydrates have to be complex carbohydrates, just the majority of them. For example, if you enjoy sandwiches on white bread, try alternating white bread with whole wheat or rye. If you dislike whole grain breads, try breads that are not 100% whole grain but offer some whole grain (at least five grams) or combinations of whole grains.

If you like cold cereal, the typical supermarket offers a wide variety of whole grain options. If you don't want to give up your sugary cereal, alternate it with whole grain cereal throughout the week. Or try filling three-quarters of the bowl with a whole grain cereal and the rest with the sugary cereal. This approach helps you satisfy the next guideline–reduce your intake of simple sugars.

Reduce Your Consumption of Simple Sugars and Sodium

Paleontology has taught us that our direct hominid ancestors (i.e., from the Paleolithic era) were a bit taller than us and had similar size brains. More important, everything we know suggests that our ancestors were quite healthy. While we don't know precisely how long they lived, it appears that when they reached old age they didn't suffer from the diseases and conditions that plague us today (e.g., diabetes, heart disease, obesity, and high blood pressure). Why? Well, their eating habits were quite different from ours.

These ancestors were omnivorous–they consumed fruits and vegetables as well as meat. More important, however, is what they didn't eat. Simple sugars (processed and refined in food plants) didn't exist. The lack of simple sugars in their diets represents a significant difference from our diets. ("Nutrition Lessons from the Stone Age - Clues to Better Eating Go Back 40,000 Years," Tufts University Health & Nutrition Letter, May 2001.) As noted earlier, fruits contain simple sugars (fructose), but the amount of calories derived from the simple sugar in fruits is limited, and fruits provide a host of vitamins and minerals.

To reduce your intake of simple sugars, you have to be able to identify which foods have a high sugar content. That part's easy. Foods that taste sweet contain large amounts of sugar. These include ice cream, chocolate, soda, cakes, pie, jam, candy, doughnuts, syrup and some fruit juices.

Soda and other sugar-laden drinks are so high in calories that you could lose weight just by eliminating them from your diet. While diet soda does not contain as much sugar as regular soda, it does have other ingredients that may adversely affect your health, such as caffeine and artificial sweeteners. But you don't have to give up soda entirely; just limit your intake. Try occasionally substituting water, an important nutrient with zero calories that is quite effective at satisfying thirst.

Just as they didn't have sugar, our Paleolithic ancestors were also deprived of salt. Natural foods, including meat, didn't go through any processing or packaging, and therefore didn't contain added salt. The lack of salt in our ancestors' diets no doubt contributed to their good health. Excess salt in the diet has been linked to high blood pressure, which can lead to heart disease, and can cause the loss of bone minerals and calcium.

Foods high in sodium include bacon, pretzels, ketchup, soy sauce, lunch meat, hot dogs, frozen meals, salted nuts, potato chips, corn chips, crackers, canned soups, salad dressing, stuffing and salami. To follow a sensible eating lifestyle, limit your intake of these and other high-sodium foods and avoid the saltshaker at meal times.

Substitute Monounsaturated and Polyunsaturated Fats for Saturated Fats

The first step in following this guideline is to limit your intake of saturated fat. The next time you go to the diner and want to order a cheeseburger, try the grilled chicken sandwich instead. Or order the hamburger and eliminate the cheese. Instead of fries, which are high in saturated fat and trans fat, order a baked potato. When buying meat in the grocery store, pick up the leaner cuts. Even fast food restaurants now offer lower-fat options. Every step you take toward reducing your saturated fat intake, however small, is a move toward adopting a sensible eating lifestyle.

Following the first guideline (increase your intake of whole grain foods) and fourth guideline (eat more fruits and vegetables) will help you cut down on the amount of saturated fat you consume. Complex carbohydrates, fruits and vegetables tend to fill you up and leave less room for additional food. If your hunger is satisfied, you will be less likely to binge on high-fat foods.

Once you reduce your saturated fat intake, you can increase your consumption of polyunsaturated and monounsaturated fat. As noted earlier, vegetable oils, such as canola, corn, olive, soybean, and sunflower oils, are high in polyunsaturated and monounsaturated fats. Use these good fats as much as possible when cooking or preparing meals. Use olive oil on your bread instead of butter. Use olive or canola oil-based dressings on your salad instead of creamy dressings. Top your sandwiches with oil and vinegar instead of mayonnaise.

Foods containing polyunsaturated fat and monounsaturated fat are just as satisfying as foods high in saturated fat, without the adverse impact on your health.

Eat More Fruits and Vegetables

You've heard it since you were a kid: "Eat your vegetables." You probably remember Popeye's muscles bulging through his skin after he ate his spinach. Mothers (and animators) everywhere can't be wrong. Fruits and vegetables are essential components of a sensible eating lifestyle.

Many of us have neglected fruits and vegetables as our reliance on fast foods and sweets for sustenance has increased due to our busy lifestyles. I've suggested to students, clients and friends that they write reminder notes to eat more fruits and vegetables and place them around the house and in their cars. This practice has enabled many of them to make a habit of eating fruits and vegetables every day.

Fruits and vegetables are carbohydrates. Fruits contain the simple sugar fructose. As stated earlier, the concentration of fructose in fruit is generally much lower than the concentration found in sugar-sweetened beverages, such as juices and sodas. Because the concentration of fructose is lower, fruits do not provide a significant number of calories. Vegetables, unlike fruits, are good sources of complex carbohydrates and therefore also satisfy the first guideline.

Different colored fruits and vegetables contain different nutrients. For example, carrots contain carotene, while bananas contain potassium. Thus eating a variety of fruits and vegetables—a palette of different colors—will provide a healthy assortment of antioxidants, vitamins and minerals.

Fruits and vegetables also tend to contain a lot of fiber, which is beneficial to your health. Some of the health benefits of fiber include reducing the risk of developing colon, rectal, breast, and ovarian cancer, heart disease, type 2 diabetes, diverticulitis, ulcerative colitis, high blood cholesterol and hemorrhoids. Due to its bulk in the digestive tract, fiber tends to fill you up. Therefore eating a high fiber diet can also help you control your weight.

Fruits and vegetables contain high levels of antioxidants, which also have many health benefits. Antioxidants found in fruits and vegetables include Vitamin C, which is found in citrus fruits, strawberries and cantaloupe; Beta-carotene, found in carrots, broccoli and sweet potatoes; and Vitamin E, found in leafy green vegetables. Antioxidants destroy free radicals in the body, which damage DNA and cell membranes. The damage that they may cause precedes certain illnesses, such as Alzheimer's disease, cardiovascular disease, Parkinson's disease, and rheumatoid arthritis.

Students will often tell me that they can't find a fruit or vegetable they like. When I press them, however, I almost always find at least one fruit or vegetable that they will tolerate or even enjoy. I suggest they try eating that particular fruit or vegetable more often. If you find only one fruit and one vegetable you are okay with, have them every day for two weeks. Becoming accustomed to eating a fruit and vegetable each day will encourage you to incorporate additional fruits and vegetables into your eating lifestyle.

Eating fruits and vegetables every day is essential to having more energy and feeling better. You can't have a sensible eating lifestyle without incorporating this practice.

Remember, adopting a sensible eating lifestyle is not about deprivation. You don't have to completely avoid the high-fat, salty and sugary foods that you enjoy. But if you limit your intake of these foods and increase your consumption of whole grains, fruits and vegetables, you're engaging in a sensible eating lifestyle. It's all about making good choices most of the time, while still allowing yourself the occasional indulgence.

Section III

Cardiovascular Endurance Training

Chapter Six

The Heart of the Matter

Remember when you could play tennis, a game of tag, or just bound up the stairs without feeling winded? Cardiovascular (C/V) endurance training, which entails regular aerobic exercise, can help maintain or restore that youthful vigor.

As you age, the maximum amount of oxygen your body can utilize (per minute) when you engage in physical activity gradually declines and fatigue sets in sooner. Based on an analysis of thirty studies evaluating the relationship between aerobic activity, aging and oxygen intake, Roy Shephard, M.D., Ph.D., at the University of Toronto, found that raising the intensity of aerobic activity not only slows the decline, but also reverses it. ("Aerobic Activity Fights Aging, Extends Independence," Tufts University Health & Nutrition Letter, July 2008).

C/V endurance training can also ward off certain medical conditions and prolong your life. Many Americans lead sedentary lifestyles, and this inactivity increases their risk of developing cardiovascular disease, suffering a heart attack, or having a stroke, according to the Centers for Disease Control and Prevention. Scientific evidence suggests that C/V endurance training will reduce the risk of heart attack and stroke.

Dr. Shephard suggested that aerobic fitness could indirectly extend indepenence by guarding against debilitating conditions such as obesity, diabetes, heart disease and stroke.

Studies also suggest that improving your cardiovascular endurance can enhance your intellectual functioning and protect you from such ailments as Alzheimer's disease. One study found that engaging in even moderate aerobic activity could significantly improve brain function. ("Fitness for Your Brain: Exercise Reverses Mental Decline," Tufts University Health & Nutrition Letter, January 2009).

Clearly, increasing your cardiovascular endurance through aerobic exercise can positively impact the length and quality of your life. Through proper C/V endurance training, your cardiovascular system will be able to adapt to changes in the intensity of your physical activities. What this means is, you'll be able to climb stairs, take longer walks, and even participate in sports without getting tired out too quickly. Just think of it as perpetual service and maintenance for your heart.

Cardiovascular System 101

To grasp the benefits of aerobic exercise, it's important to understand the basic functioning of your C/V system. So let's take a trip back to biology class and review. The C/V system is made up of the heart, blood vessels, lungs and blood. Blood containing oxygen leaves your heart, travels throughout your body dropping off that oxygen to your organs and tissues, picks up oxygen in your lungs, and returns to the heart to be pumped out all over again.

As you can see, the heart is the hub of this intricate transportation system. The heart is a muscle (cardiac muscle). Each type of muscle causes movement of some kind. The heart causes blood to move. Contractions of cardiac muscle are called beats. In between beats, the heart rests.

The left side of the heart pumps oxygenated blood (blood containing oxygen) into the largest artery, the aorta, which branches off into smaller vessels so that the blood can be delivered all around the body. Veins carry blood without oxygen back to the right side of the heart. It is then pumped to the lungs where carbon dioxide is exchanged for oxygen. Oxygen enters the lungs when we inhale air, and carbon dioxide is expelled when we exhale.

Increasing Cardiovascular Endurance Through Aerobic Exercise

C/V endurance training can strengthen your heart and increase the efficiency of your cardiovascular system, enabling you to sustain physical activity for longer periods of time and delay the onset of fatigue.

Aerobic (with oxygen) exercise is a physical activity that is continuous (as opposed to stop and go). The body uses oxygen as its primary source of energy for these activities. The following activities would be considered aerobic: jogging, walking, cross country skiing, non-competitive cycling and swimming. (Anaerobic exercise, such as weight training, is physical activity that is non-continuous and uses glucose, not oxygen, as the primary source of energy.)

Kenneth H. Cooper, M.D., M.P.H., known as the "father of aerobics," shifted the emphasis from disease treatment to disease prevention through aerobic exercise. He introduced the term in his first book, titled *Aerobics*, back in 1968. Dr. Cooper ignited a revolution by advocating the pursuit of C/V fitness and extolling the importance of regular aerobic exercise.

Aerobic exercise benefits your C/V system by improving its ability to use oxygen. It causes the heart to beat faster, delivering more oxygen rich blood and nutrients around your body. As your heart becomes stronger, it can produce more forceful contractions, which pump more blood with each beat. This results in a slower heart rate and longer rest periods between heart beats. Therefore, a trained cardiovascular system can adapt to increases in the intensity of your physical activity by supplying muscles with more oxygenated blood. Dr. Cooper referred to the physiological benefits of aerobic exercise as the "training effect."

A Word of Caution

Many of my clients have expressed concern that engaging in aerobic exercise will lead to a heart attack. They often cite the case of Jim Fixx, the iconic runner and fitness guru who seemed to be in excellent cardiovascular shape but died of a heart attack while jogging. But it wasn't Fixx's C/V training regimen that killed him. In fact, his training probably extended his life. It was his risk factors that led to his death, including arteriosclerosis (clogged arteries), which is the underlying cause of heart attacks. The autopsy showed that all three of his coronary arteries were blocked. Despite Fixx's family medical history (his father had his first heart attack at the age of 35 and died of a heart attack at 43), Fixx didn't have a regular physician or undergo a routine physical exam.

You do occasionally hear of individuals who suffer heart attacks while engaging in strenuous aerobic activity. While these instances are rare, they often involve individuals who are not in good enough physical shape to engage in rigorous physical activity. This is why I advise my clients and students to consult their physicians before beginning a new exercise program or increasing the intensity of their current exercise regimen. I suggest you do the same. You have to make sure that you're fit enough to engage in the C/V program you're planning to undertake. If you're not in proper physical condition, you have to start off slowly and progress at your own pace. Your doctor will be able to advise you on what physical activities are safe and appropriate for you.

Chapter Seven

The Path to Cardiovascular Fitness

Now that you know the benefits of C/V endurance training, let's talk about how you can develop an effective aerobic exercise regimen. To increase your C/V endurance, you have to do the following:

- Increase your heart rate.
- Keep it elevated for a period of time.
- Engage in aerobic exercise regularly.

In this chapter, I'll explain how to accomplish these three elements of C/V endurance training. I will also discuss how you can maintain your momentum and continue to improve your C/V endurance by increasing the intensity, duration and frequency of your training program.

Increasing Your Heart Rate

Any aerobic activity will increase your heart rate. Select one that you like because you'll be more likely to stick with your exercise regimen if you enjoy it. You can engage in aerobic activity inside or outside, with or without equipment. The activity you choose should meet the following criteria: (1) you're familiar with it; (2) you're physically able to do it; (3) it's continuous; (4) it's non-competitive. Examples of aerobic activity include the following:

- Walking, jogging or running on a treadmill, on an inside track, on an outside track, in a recreational area or park, around your block or neighborhood.
- Step-ups (stepping up and down on the bottom step of a stairway inside or outside your home, or on equipment designed for step-ups).
- Swimming laps in an indoor or outdoor pool.
- Riding your bicycle around the block, on a bike trail, or on a scenic tour.
- Riding a stationary bicycle in your home or at the gym.
- Roller blading or roller skating.
- Cross country skiing.

How High Should My Heart Rate Be?

To benefit from aerobic exercise, you must get your heart rate into a specific range known as your target zone (TZ). I suggest you use 50% to 85% of your maximum heart rate (MHR) as your TZ.

How Do I Calculate My Target Zone?

To calculate your TZ, you first need to know your MHR. The fastest a heart can beat is 220 beats per minute. Your MHR decreases by about one beat per minute each year as you age. If you subtract your age from 220, you will have your MHR.

For example, if you are fifty years old, your MHR will be 220 - 50 = 170 beats per minute (BPM).

Now that you know your MHR, you're ready to calculate your TZ. The lower end of your TZ is 50% of your MHR, so multiply your MHR by 0.50. The upper end of your TZ is 85% of your MHR, so multiply your MHR by 0.85.

If you're fifty years old, the lower end of your TZ would be 170 x 0.50 = 85 BPM. The upper end would be 170 x 0.85 = 144.5 BPM. So to reach your TZ, you will have to get your heart rate up to at least 85 BPM, but it's not necessary to exceed 144.5 BPM.

Use the following table to calculate your own TZ:

My Target Zone (TZ)
220 - _____ (your age) = _____ (your MHR)
0.50 x _____ (your MHR) = _____ (lower end of TZ)
0.85 x _____ (your MHR) = _____ (upper end of TZ)
TZ = _____ to _____

How Do I Monitor My Heart Rate?

Now that you know your TZ, you have to learn how to determine whether your heart rate is in this range. You can monitor your heart rate in one of two ways: (1) manually taking your pulse, or (2) using an electronic monitoring device.

Every time your heart beats you can feel a pulse in certain arteries that lie close to the surface of the skin. The most commonly used sites are the groove in your wrist just below the base of your thumb and on either side of your neck just below the lower jaw bone near the edge of your windpipe. Don't take your pulse with your thumb because it has a pulse of its own; use your index and middle fingers. Don't press too hard or you may not be able to find or feel your pulse.

Heart rate is usually measured by counting the number of beats per minute (BPM). However, it's not necessary to count the number of beats for a full sixty seconds. You can count the number of beats, for example, for ten seconds and multiply by six, or count for fifteen seconds and multiply by four.

It can be difficult to take your pulse while engaged in an aerobic activity (to determine whether you're in your TZ). It's also tricky to take it after your workout because one pulse may seem to go into the next or your pulse may be erratic (i.e., three quick beats and a subsequent skipped beat). You can try counting for thirty seconds or longer, or try taking your pulse two or three times in a row.

Using an electronic heart rate monitoring device can alleviate the problems associated with taking your pulse manually during and after a workout. Aerobic exercise equipment often contains sensors that will display your heart rate on the monitor or screen. You can also purchase a stand-alone heart monitoring device. These devices typically require you to wear a chest strap, which has electrodes that go over your heart. Your pulse rate is transmitted via radio signals to a watch on your wrist. Many of these devices allow you to program in the upper and lower limits of your TZ. The watch will beep when you are below the lower limit or above the upper limit.

How Fast Should I Enter and Exit My Target Zone?

You should always gradually get your heart rate up into your TZ. You should begin your cardiovascular workout with a five-minute "warm-up" period to get your heart beating a little faster. During your warm-up, gradually increase the intensity of your activity incrementally for five minutes. The intensity is determined by speed and elevation/resistance. If you're using a stationary bike or elliptical, the intensity is based on the level of resistance you select and the speed at which you pedal. On a treadmill, the level of elevation and the speed at which you walk, jog or run determine the intensity.

Let's use the treadmill as an example. Start out by walking slowly with no elevation. Alternately increase the speed and elevation gradually until you approach the intensity levels that will get you into your TZ. Never start walking at your maximum speed and elevation immediately because it can abruptly raise your blood pressure.

Along the same lines, you must incorporate a five-minute "cool-down" period at the end of your workout. During the cool-down, slowly bring your heart rate back down. Never abruptly stop your activity. For example, if you've been walking briskly or running on the treadmill at an elevation, gradually decrease your speed to a slow pace and your elevation to zero during the last five minutes of your workout.

Did I Work Hard Enough or Too Hard?

When you have completed thirty minutes of aerobic exercise, monitor your heart rate. If your heart rate is below the lower end of your TZ, you didn't work hard enough. If your heart rate exceeds the upper end of your TZ, you worked much too hard. If you determine your heart rate is not within your TZ, adjust the intensity of your workout the next time.

While not working hard enough will limit the effectiveness of your workout, working too hard can be dangerous. Instinct may cause you to slow down too quickly or stop too abruptly instead of gradually and incrementally slowing (cooling) down. This practice wreaks havoc with your blood pressure and can cause lightheadedness, dizziness and nausea.

Important Medical Considerations

As noted earlier, it is prudent to consult your physician before beginning any exercise program or participating in any competitive physical activity. Your medical and physical limitations and medical history may influence the intensity of your workouts and your TZ. In particular, if you've had a heart attack or have any type of cardiovascular disease or respiratory illness, ask your physician, cardiologist or pulmonary specialist what your MHR is and what your TZ should be.

If your heart rate goes directly to the upper end of your TZ when you start warming up, exceeds the upper end of your TZ, becomes unusually rapid, or doesn't slow down within five minutes after you stop exercising, clearly your heart is untrained and your C/V system is not working efficiently. This scenario is not unusual, especially for people who are just starting a C/V endurance training program for the first time. You should visit your physician before engaging in aerobic exercise again.

If you experience any of the following symptoms while exercising—lightheadedness, nausea, dizziness, chest pain, or tightness in your chest—you should STOP exercising immediately and seek medical attention. And you should undergo a complete physical before you engage in any type of exercise again. You should also visit your doctor if you injure yourself while exercising. Don't try to work through the pain or self medicate.

Keeping Your Heart Rate Elevated

I suggest you keep your heart rate in its TZ for twenty minutes. Including your five-minute warm-up and five-minute cool-down, your entire workout will take thirty minutes. I've found this duration works well for most people at various points on the fitness continuum. But if you're at either end of the spectrum—you're highly trained or you've never engaged in any type of exercise—you may need to vary this duration, depending on the advice of your physician and how you feel during the workout. And just as your medical or physical limitations will influence the intensity of your workout, they will also play a role in the duration and frequency of them.

If you're engaging in C/V endurance training for the first time or resuming your training after a long hiatus (months or years), it's essential that you gradually and comfortably progress at your own pace. For example, if you're out of breath after walking on a treadmill for ten minutes, don't push for twenty at this point in your training. Try walking a minute or two longer the next time.

Engaging in Aerobic Activity Regularly

I suggest engaging in aerobic exercise three to four times per week. But again, the frequency of your workouts will depend on your medical and physical limitations and your doctor's advice.

What it all comes down to is this: to increase your C/V endurance, you need to get your heart rate into its TZ and keep it there for twenty minutes three to four times per week.

How Do I Monitor My Progress?

Three factors will indicate improvements in cardiovascular endurance:

(1) The intensity of your current workout no longer gets you into your TZ.

This means your heart is working more efficiently.

(2) The time it takes your heart to return to its pre-activity rate ("recovery rate") has decreased.

It will take you less and less time to recover as you continue your training. Being able to speak and breathe normally soon after completing your workouts (up to about ten minutes) are also positive signs.

(3) Your "resting heart rate" (RHR) has decreased.

As a general rule, the lower your RHR is, the more efficiently your cardiovascular system is functioning. To determine your RHR, monitor your heart rate when you are calm and not exerting yourself (i.e., after sitting for between ten and twenty minutes). Technically, your heart rate based on this method may be somewhat higher than your true RHR. If you want a more accurate measure, take your pulse before getting out of bed for three mornings. The average of the three is your true RHR.

Maintaining Your Momentum

If you've made considerable progress in improving your C/V endurance and your workout no longer gets you into your TZ, it's time to increase the intensity of your workouts. But keep the duration and frequency constant (thirty minutes three to four times a week).

Increase the Intensity

To increase the intensity of your workouts, increase your speed and/or resistance/elevation. Later in the chapter, you'll learn how you can use Interchangeable Aerobic Training (IAT) and pre-set programs to increase the intensity of your activity. You can also try using a different piece of aerobic exercise equipment. But start out with slow speeds, light resistances and slight elevations until you get comfortable with it.

Increase the Frequency

Engaging in a thirty-minute cardio workout three times a week is sufficient. But if you have the time, you can add a fourth cardio workout if you prefer.

Increase the Duration

If you have the time, you can increase the duration of your cardio workouts. However, I strongly suggest you stick to a thirty-minute cardio workout if you do it directly before one of your weight training sessions. You can increase the duration beyond thirty minutes on a day that you're not weight training. (Weight training is covered in Section IV, Muscle Strength and Endurance Training.)

In general, however, I do not recommend increasing the amount of time spent doing any one of the three exercise components of The Awesome Foursome (C/V endurance training, muscle strength and endurance training, static stretching). Usually, increasing the duration of one takes time and energy away from the other two. More important, you may increase the risk of injuries such as sprains and strains. For example, you may be so exhausted from your cardio workout that you rush through your weight training workout or eliminate your stretching.

A Word About Weight Loss

Many people do aerobic exercise for the sole purpose of burning calories and losing weight. It may even be the only one of the three exercise components of The Awesome Foursome that they do. Indeed, studies have shown that aerobic activity does burn calories, cause weight loss, and even suppresses your appetite. Still, the most effective way to lose weight is to engage in all four components of The Awesome Foursome.

After reading the section on sensible eating, you understand the role caloric intake plays in weight gain. But when you read the following section on muscular strength and endurance, you'll see that weight training also causes weight loss, burns calories and fat, and helps to control your weight. Both aerobic exercise and weight training cause your body to burn calories during as well as after your workouts. Thus you're going to burn more calories by engaging in both aerobic exercise and weight training. More important, you're attaining the health and fitness benefits of both.

Chapter Eight

The Scoop on Aerobic Exercise Equipment

While you can jog, ride your bike, or swim laps to increase your C/V endurance, you also have the option of purchasing a piece of aerobic exercise equipment or using one at a fitness club. In this chapter I'll explain how to use the following pieces of equipment safely and effectively: the treadmill, stationary bike, elliptical, stepper and rowing machine. I'll also provide you with options for varying your workouts.

Equipment Options

Aerobic exercise involves making repetitive movements at various intensity levels for various durations of time. The pieces of equipment described here allow you to accomplish this. I've personally used all of these pieces and have evaluated them based on four primary factors: safety, effectiveness, efficiency and user-friendliness.

Treadmill

You can walk, run or jog on a treadmill. You can vary the elevation and speed of the treadmill to adjust the intensity of your workouts. Most people just adjust the speed and never use the elevation. But raising the elevation on a treadmill is an effective way to increase your heart rate. It's harder to walk or run up a hill than on level ground because it's more work for your leg muscles and your C/V system.

Almost all treadmills start at a minimum tread belt speed of 0.5 miles per hour (MPH). You can adjust the speed in tenth of a mile increments and elevation in 1% increments.

If you're using a treadmill for the first time, you may start out walking faster than the tread belt when it's moving at slow speeds, and slower than the belt when it's moving at faster speeds. Adjust your pace to the speed of the belt, and soon you'll be in sync with it.

Don't constantly hold on to the front rails of the treadmill unless you have a medical/physical reason to do so. You can grasp the front rail with one or both hands to maintain your balance whenever necessary. However, once you are comfortable, you should walk, jog or run without holding on to the front rail. When you engage in these activities outside, you don't hold on to anything. More important, holding on keeps your heart rate down. Also, you'll burn far fewer calories if you hold on to the rail because you're not working as hard.

When walking, jogging or running on the treadmill, maintain good posture (don't slouch).

Stationary Bike

Stationary bikes come in two varieties: upright and semi-recumbent. The upright stationary bike is modeled after a traditional bicycle. The semi-recumbent bike requires you to sit on a more traditional seat (with a back) and extend your legs out in front of you as opposed to vertically. If you have a lower back problem, I would urge you to try a semi-recumbent stationary bike because it offers back support. The seat has a handle on each side to grasp for stability, and is more comfortable than those on upright stationary bikes.

Stationary bikes have two intensity variables: speed of pedaling and resistance to pedaling.

Before you start, you have to adjust the seat height to accommodate you. To do this on an upright bike, sit on the bike, put one foot on the lower pedal, and adjust the seat height so that the bend in that leg is just enough to keep your foot comfortably anchored on the pedal. If the seat is too low, your legs will be bent too much and they will tire quickly. If the seat is too high, you'll have to strain to keep your feet in contact with the pedals.

On the semi-recumbent bike, your legs extend out in front of you at a slight downward angle so that when your feet are in the pedals, they are below the seat height. The seat can be adjusted by moving it forward or backward. Before you start, place one foot in the pedal furthest away from you and adjust the seat so that the bend in that leg is enough to keep your foot anchored in the pedal.

Elliptical

Elliptical machines provide for a natural walking, jogging or running motion. I like the natural movement pattern of the elliptical and the ability to adjust my speed by simply pedaling faster or slower. An advantage of the elliptical machine is it allows you to use both your upper and lower body muscles, intensifying your workout.

An elliptical machine has two intensity variables: speed of pedaling (to simulate walking, jogging and running), and resistance to pedaling.

Ellipticals have long pedals for your feet and two vertical handle bars that you alternately push forward and pull back. Using the vertical handlebars increases intensity. The movement is similar to the arm swing when you walk, jog or run, and is in sync with your pedaling. If you don't want to use the vertical handlebars, you can hold on to a fixed front rail.

Stride lengths on ellipticals can be shortened or lengthened (automatically) by inches to accommodate your height and leg length. This is important because you want to ensure you go through a full range of motion, but you don't want to stride too far. In either case, the effectiveness and efficiency of the movement is constrained, and the potential for injury is heightened.

Stepper

Steppers require you to step straight up and down onto different pedals against resistance. You can execute the stepping motion with your entire foot or only the balls of your feet on the pedals. The two intensity variables are speed and resistance.

If you're just starting out with a C/V endurance training program or you have not followed one for three months or more, I would not recommend the stepper. It's not a natural movement. When walking, jogging or running, you step out, but on a straight (up and down) stepper, you're stepping straight down and coming straight up. In addition, stepping this way against resistance repetitively can strain leg muscles, and stress the hips, lower back, knees and ankles.

Rowing Machine

Individuals who use rowing machines tend to be experienced competitive rowers, or they enjoy recreational rowing. If you have not engaged in C/V endurance training for three months or more or have never rowed a boat, I would not recommend a rowing machine. Rowing is an intense aerobic activity because it requires you to use your upper and lower body muscles, and the rhythmic and coordinated movement pattern requires practice. In addition, the seats don't have backs, so you run the risk of hyper-extending your lower back (beyond a 90 degree angle with your hips).

To use a rowing machine, you move yourself back and forth on tracks using your arms and legs. Always keep your hips and back at a 90 degree angle. When you pull the bar or row handle toward your abdomen, keep your elbows close to your sides. Flaring your elbows out can put a strain on your shoulders. When you extend your arms, avoid locking out your elbows (maintain a slight bend in your arms). Also avoid hyper-extending your knees when you push back with your legs.

The resistance and speed variables on rowing machines have a reciprocal relationship. The faster you pull the row bar toward your abdomen, the easier it is to pull. Conversely, the slower you pull the row bar, the harder it is to pull. To manually adjust the resistance on some of the commercial rowing machines, you have to take one or both hands off of the row handle and stop the rowing motion. This breaks the continuity of a C/V endurance workout.

Workout Options

Pre-Set Programs

Most pieces of aerobic equipment have pre-set programs that automatically change the speed and resistance during your workout. You usually have three or four primary programs to choose from, but each has several levels of intensity, giving you a wide range of options. You can choose levels in each of the primary programs that accommodate your current level of fitness and then select higher intensity level programs as you progress. Some of the programs have names, such as "fat burning" or "weight loss." As noted earlier, aerobic exercise does burn calories and leads to weight loss. But the most efficient way to get healthy and fit is to engage in all four components of The Awesome Foursome.

I would suggest starting out with low intensity programs and progressing to higher intensity options in each of the primary programs. Pre-set programs are convenient and offer a variety of challenges as you go through your cardiovascular endurance training.

Interchangeable Aerobic Training (IAT)

I developed the Interchangeable Aerobic Training (IAT) approach to C/V workouts while using my first treadmill, which didn't offer pre-set programs. I found that using this approach made my workouts more effective, as well as more interesting. You can use IAT on any aerobic piece of equipment, including those that have pre-set programs.

IAT involves alternately changing the two intensity variables (speed and resistance/elevation) for different lengths of time. You increase or decrease each variable one at a time—never at the same time. Making changes manually—instead of using a pre-set program—eliminates the restrictions on the number of changes you can make and removes constraints on the duration of each change. For example, if you're using a treadmill, increase the elevation while walking or jogging. When you're running, decrease the elevation. Similarly, on stationary bikes or ellipticals, pedal faster at lower resistances, and slower at higher resistances.

If you're just starting out, IAT is a great way for you to get into C/V endurance training because you're in complete control of the workouts and you can progress at your own pace. If you've been using pre-set programs, IAT will be a challenging change of pace that allows you to manually create programs that advance your progress. In any case, you may need a few trial-and-error sessions to determine which speeds and intensity levels get you into your TZ.

The IAT concept is more familiar to you than you may think. Chances are, you've already experienced your body's response to different challenges to your C/V system. Have you ever walked or jogged up and down hills? You probably adjusted your speed based on the steepness and length of the hills. Walking on a level surface rapidly and walking up a hill more slowly pose different challenges to your C/V system.

In the same way, IAT allows you to challenge yourself (and your heart) in different ways by adjusting the two intensity variables alternately. When you adjust (increase or decrease) the intensity variables, pay attention to how you feel. Do you find it more difficult to move at a higher speed or at a higher level of resistance/elevation? If you find that moving faster is more challenging than moving at a higher resistance, then spend more time at faster speeds. Conversely, if you find that moving against higher resistances is more challenging, then spend more time at higher resistances.

Just about all physical activities require stop and go movements and short and long bursts of speed and power. Your heart has to be trained to acclimate to varying levels of intensity and be efficient enough to take advantage of low intensity moments to rest. IAT and pre-set programs provide the variability to increase cardiovascular endurance. Maintaining the same speed and resistance throughout your C/V workouts does not provide the necessary variability.

Cross Training

To keep your C/V workouts fresh and challenging, try using two different pieces of aerobic exercise equipment during each training session. This concept is called cross training.

Any two of the pieces discussed here can be used within the same thirty-minute C/V endurance workout. Use one piece for fifteen minutes and the other for fifteen minutes. Do your five-minute warm-up and continue for ten minutes on one piece of equipment. Move on to the other piece of equipment for the next ten minutes, finishing with a five-minute cool-down. You can also use a different piece of equipment for each of the week's three cardio workouts.

Cross training challenges your C/V system because it requires you to engage in different movement patterns during your workouts and allows you to alter intensity levels in a variety of ways. An added benefit of cross training is that it may make your workouts more interesting and enjoyable.

Section IV

Muscle Strength and Endurance Training

Chapter Nine

The Might of Muscles

If you adopt a sensible eating lifestyle and engage in aerobic exercise regularly, you will most likely lose weight (if that's your goal) or maintain your weight. But you will not change the shape of your body. Only muscle strength and endurance training, otherwise known as weight training, will do that. In fact, muscles that are strong and toned burn more calories even when at rest than do muscles that are not developed.

This section will arm you with the information you need to use weight-training machines safely and properly. After reading this section, you'll be able to walk into any gym or fitness store, and you won't feel intimidated by the machines. I'll give you a basic overview of weight training, a detailed description of exercises you should do for a total body workout, and a selection of workout routines.

But first let's talk about how muscles work and why building muscle strength and endurance is beneficial.

Muscular Physiology 101

When muscles contract, they move one bone closer to another bone. The joint is where the two bones meet and movement takes place (e.g., elbow, knee, hip, shoulder). Ligaments hold two bones together at joints. Different types of joints allow different movements and ranges of motion (ROM). The elbow and knee are "hinge" joints, which allow a joint to bend and straighten only (move back and forth like a door). The shoulder and hip are "ball and socket" joints, which allow movement in any direction, including around in a circle. The wrist and ankle are "gliding" joints, which allow a limited ROM (sliding, twisting, circular). Muscles are not directly attached to the bones; they're attached by connective tissue called tendons. Cartilage is also connective tissue that covers the ends of bones at the joints. It serves as a cushion, or shock absorber, to prevent bone on bone friction.

Muscles that bend (flex) limbs are called flexor muscles. Muscles that straighten (lengthen or extend) limbs are called extensor muscles. For example, the quadriceps muscles in the front of the thighs (the "kicking muscles") are extensor muscles because they extend or straighten the legs at the knee joints. The hamstrings in the back of the legs are flexor muscles because they bend or flex the legs at the knee joints.

As you can see from the example above, muscles work in pairs. When one muscle contracts (shortens), the other one of the pair extends (lengthens). Here's another example: the triceps muscles in the back of the upper arms (the "throwing muscles") are extensor muscles because they extend or straighten the arms at the elbows. The biceps muscles in the front of the upper arms are flexor muscles because they bend or flex the arms at the elbows.

To improve your performance in any physical activity and reduce the potential for injury, the strength of your muscles that work in pairs should be balanced. That doesn't mean you should be able to lift the same amount of weight with each muscle. It means the strength of each relative to its size should be the same. You don't want to work muscles selectively or randomly because this can cause strength imbalances, a leading cause of orthopedic injuries, such as sprains, strains and tears. When tendons and muscles are strained (stretched or torn), movement is impaired and painful. Unlike muscles and tendons, ligaments are not elastic. When ligaments are sprained (stretched or torn), they will heal, but they will not return to their original length, compromising the joint.

Your muscles, tendons, ligaments, cartilage and bones must be structurally and functionally sound for proper movement to take place at the joints. Muscle strength and endurance training will improve the efficiency, strength and power of your movements. Efficient movement will also significantly reduce your susceptibility to injury.

Benefits of Muscle Strength and Endurance Training

Increasing your muscle strength and endurance will not only improve your performance in sports and other physical recreational activities, but it will also make your daily activities easier, such as carrying groceries, playing with your children or grandchildren, pushing a stroller, or doing housework. You'll also find that strenuous physical activities, such as chopping wood, moving furniture and carrying heavy items, will be easier. Increased muscle strength and endurance will allow you to perform all of these activities more efficiently, effectively and for longer periods of time, and reduce your risk of injury.

As you get older, maintaining muscle strength and endurance is particularly important. Muscles atrophy from nonuse. Weight training will enable you to maintain muscle strength and endurance, good balance, and pain-free full ranges of motion around joints.

Performing weight-bearing exercises also strengthens bones, which can become brittle with age. Because weight-bearing exercises limit or prevent bone loss, weight training can help protect you from osteoporosis.

If you have hypertension (high blood pressure) or you're at risk for the condition, weight training can help. According to the Strength and Conditioning Journal, weight training makes it possible for people to become more physically active, which helps control or prevent high blood pressure ("Hypertension and Resistance Training," Strength and Conditioning Journal, February 2009.)

Through strength and endurance training, you'll be able to perform activities that were previously challenging, and you'll improve the quality of your life.

A Word of Caution

As I mentioned in the previous section, it's imperative that you consult your doctor before beginning a new exercise program or changing your current regimen. Before you start doing the exercises suggested in this section, make an appointment to see your physician. If you have certain medical or physical conditions or you're taking medication, it may not be advisable for you to do some of the exercises or workouts. Or, your doctor or specialist (e.g., your cardiologist or orthopedist) may recommend some adaptations.

Chapter Ten

Getting Started: Weight Training Basics

Building Blocks of Your Workout Routine

Repetitions (Reps)

The first movement of any weight-training exercise is called a "positive" or "concentric" contraction. The second movement is called a "negative" or "eccentric" contraction. Both movements are equally important to a muscle's development.

Every time you do both the positive and negative movements, you've done one "repetition" or rep. Positive reps should take about four seconds to complete, and negative reps about five or six seconds.

Sets

A specific number of repetitions is called a "set." A commonly accepted practice is to do multiple sets—typically three, but five or ten is not unusual. However, recent studies show that one-set workouts are equally effective. One-set workouts are efficient because they take less time, enabling you to work at higher intensity levels without getting tired. One-set workouts are also safer and reduce the risk of injury because the number of reps is significantly decreased.

For these reasons, I recommend you do only one set for each exercise. An important concept known as "momentary failure" is the basis for this recommendation. When you lift weights you're inducing the momentary failure of muscles. When a muscle reaches momentary failure, you experience a sensation often referred to as "the burn." It's a sore, tired or uncomfortable feeling in your muscles. The burn is a reaction to the microscopic tearing of muscle fibers. The body repairs the microscopic muscle tears caused by momentary failure during your rest period (discussed later in this chapter). The repair process increases the size and strength of muscles in small increments. When you induce momentary failure in one set you've achieved the benefit of that exercise.

Not only are one-set workouts more efficient because they're less time-consuming, they're also safer. When enough fibers are torn, the muscle can no longer forcefully contract. Going beyond the burn and doing another rep will increase your risk of injury. You should stop when you feel the burn.

Keep in mind, as you progress, increasing the intensity of your workouts will be more effective than increasing the number of sets or reps you do. I discuss how you can increase the intensity of your workouts later in Chapter Twelve.

Weights

Before I can explain how to determine the amount of weight you should lift for each exercise, you need to understand the five characteristics of muscles:

- **Strength** determines how much weight you can lift, push or pull. Strength is based on the amount of force muscles can produce or how forcefully they can contract and cause movement against resistance.
- **Power** is the speed at which you can lift, push or pull a heavy weight. It's a function of time.
- **Local muscular endurance** refers to the length of time a muscle can keep contracting and causing movement before it succumbs to fatigue.
- **Tone** refers to the degree of firmness and tension in muscles. Toned muscles engage in what I call "multiple mini contractions" twenty-four hours a day. This activity keeps muscles in a constant state of readiness, which enables them to contract and cause movement in an instant.
- **Definition** refers to the contours or outline of muscles (i.e., the two parts of the biceps muscles are clearly defined).

Weight training will help you develop three of these characteristics: strength, power, and local muscular endurance. Lifting weights alone will not develop tone or definition. The factor that influences the tone and definition of your muscles is your body's percentage of lean body mass (muscle) compared to your body's percentage of excess fat. The more excess fat that covers up a muscle, the less visible its contours are. Excess fat also obscures the tight look associated with tone. When you lower your percentage of excess fat and build muscle, definition is enhanced and muscles will look more firm (toned). As noted earlier, a sensible eating lifestyle combined with a regular exercise regimen will help you control your weight.

So how can you develop strength, power and local muscular endurance through weight training?

In general, to increase strength and power, use heavier weights and do fewer reps. Strength and power are highly related. As muscles become stronger, they can apply more force and therefore move a weight at higher speeds.

To increase local muscular endurance, use lighter weights and do more reps.

But how do you determine how much weight to lift and how many reps to do for each exercise?

To increase strength, find a weight for each exercise that you can lift between four and eight times. In other words, you should be able to do at least four reps without feeling the burn or straining. If you feel the burn and start to strain between the fifth and eighth rep, the weight is appropriate. As noted earlier, stop doing reps when you feel the burn and have to strain to do a rep.

To increase local muscular endurance, find a weight for each exercise that you can lift between fourteen and eighteen times. You should be able to do at least fourteen reps without feeling the burn or straining, but no more than eighteen reps.

If you're just starting out, it may take a few trial and error sessions to determine the appropriate amounts of weight you should lift for each exercise. Do a couple of reps with different amounts of weight. Ask yourself the following questions: "At what point did I feel the burn?" "Could I have done more reps?" "Did I strain to do four or five with proper form?" (Form is discussed later in this chapter.)

As you increase strength and local muscular endurance over a period of weeks or months, you will have to adjust the amounts of weight you use, and possibly the numbers of reps you do.

It's important that you increase both strength and local muscular endurance. But you can't do both in the same workout. I recommend alternating, on a regular basis, between strength workouts and local muscular endurance workouts to achieve the benefits of both.

Rest Period

One of the cardinal rules in weight training is to NEVER work the same muscle two days in a row. Everyone needs at least twenty-four hours of rest between workouts. Many of us need two or three days of rest between workouts.

Rest periods are just as important as the workouts. During rest periods the body repairs the microscopic muscle tears caused by momentary failure. The repair process increases the size and strength of muscles in small increments. The cumulative effect over a period of weeks, months and years is stronger muscles that will resist fatigue. If you keep breaking down muscles without giving the body a chance to repair them, you'll achieve little to no muscle development and greatly increase your potential for injury.

Proper Form Is Essential

To work out safely and achieve results, you must adhere to proper form. Proper form enables you to "isolate" the muscle you're working (i.e., only that muscle is contracting and lifting the weight). If you're not adhering to proper form, it's likely that other muscles are helping, and the targeted muscle will be cheated out of doing 100% of the work. For example, proper form for two-arm biceps curls requires that you don't move your elbows away from your sides. If your elbows lose contact with your sides by moving forward and up, your shoulder muscles are helping the biceps muscles do the curls.

Not only is proper form effective, it also can prevent injuries. I believe that a high percentage of injuries, such as sprains and strains, that are sustained playing sports are related to the lack of proper form while weight training. In other words, you are more susceptible to injuries while engaging in physical activity if you don't adhere to proper form while weight training. First, you predispose your body to injuries when you engage in potentially damaging movements, such as locking out joints. In addition, you're not achieving adequate muscle development, which would enable your body to avoid injuries.

To ensure you're using proper form when weight training, adhere to the following guidelines:

- **Do every exercise slowly and smoothly.** Avoid herky-jerky movements.
- **Go through a full range of motion (ROM).** A complete range of

motion is the distance between the point where the muscles come under tension to the point just before rest.

- **Don't "rest" the muscle you're working.** If the weights that you're lifting (on the positive rep) touch the top plate of the weight stack on the way down (on the negative rep), the muscle is no longer under tension and it rests. Keep the contractions going throughout every repetition by momentarily pausing when there is a slight bend in the joints. This increases the time that the muscles are under tension, leading to greater increases in strength and local muscular endurance. If you're new to weight training, you may have to stare at the weight plates on the machine to make sure they don't touch.
- **Never lock out a joint** because this can damage cartilage, muscles, tendons and bones. Locking out means that you have fully extended your arms or legs and couldn't physically go any further. Always stop when the joint is slightly bent.
- **Keep your wrists in a "neutral position."** If you're using bars, handles or other accessories for upper body exercises, proper form dictates that the top of your hand and the top of your forearm make a straight line. There is no bend in your wrist. Your wrists must remain in this position when you're doing all but two of the exercises described (wrist curls and reverse wrist curls).
- **Control negative reps.** Doing fast, uncontrolled negative reps is a common practice and one of the most egregious examples of improper form. You have to control the weight in both directions—on the positive rep and the negative rep. If you do a slow and controlled positive rep but then allow gravity to bring down the weight plates, you're not in control of the weight. The muscle did

only half of the work, and you will likely lock out the joints.

Don't Forget to Breath

You may think this advice is obvious, but I've seen people channel so much of their focus into their positive reps that they hold their breath. But proper breathing is critical for effective and safe weight training. If you find it difficult to breath normally while lifting weights, I suggest the following: exhale lightly on the positive rep, and inhale on the negative rep. You want to get rid of carbon dioxide during the positive rep and take in oxygen during the negative rep. The exhalation should be light because forceful exhalations can cause you to become light-headed and dizzy. Your breathing should be rhythmical and remain in sync with your positive and negative reps.

Free Weights vs. Machines

Research shows that free weights and weight-training machines are equally effective at building strength. In general, I recommend using machines to do all of the exercises described in the next chapter, except for the abdominal exercises, which can be done on a mat. I find machines to be easier and more convenient to use than free weights. However, if you've been working out with free weights and have achieved positive results, I encourage you to continue to do so.

Using Weight-training Machines

Gyms and fitness centers have single-station machines, multi-station machines, and free-standing units. A single-station machine has only one weight stack. It allows one person at a time to do one particular exercise (e.g., bench press machine). Multi-station machines have three or four weight stacks and allow up to four people to work out simultaneously.

Single-station machines usually have signs that show a picture of the muscle the machine works, along with written instructions for how to use the machine. On multi-station machines, a wide variety of accessories/specialty bars and handles are available to attach to upper and lower pulleys. Make sure you take up the slack in the cables to ensure that you will have tension immediately when starting the first positive rep, allowing you to maintain muscle contraction throughout the full ROM of every rep. For example, when you're facing the weight plates, if you feel tension immediately when starting the positive rep, you're standing in the correct spot. If you feel slack in the cable, move back a bit.

To change the amount of weight you'll be lifting for each exercise, you place an "L" shaped pin into a weight plate on the stack.

Most single-station machines have seats, as do some stations on multi-station machines. Seats adjust up and down to accommodate your height. When sitting for an exercise on a single-station machine, make sure your hips are all the way back in the seat, forming a 90 degree angle with your back and hips. Keeping your back against the back support pad will ensure that your back is straight and supported. You don't want to slouch or lean forward.

If you prefer to work out at home, home gyms are available. These compact units have one weight stack, usually with ten pound plates totaling about 200 pounds, and are available in a variety of configurations. They have high and low pulleys, a vertical bench press and butterfly station, a leg extension/leg curl station, adjustable seats and seat backs, and attachments, such as a leg press station.

Warming Up, Cooling Down

Your weight-training workout must always begin with a warm-up. It's essential that you "warm up" your muscles before working them to avoid injury. Engaging in any of the aerobic exercises discussed in the previous section for five to ten minutes will serve as an adequate warm-up. Remember to gradually increase the intensity of the aerobic activity. You can, of course, do a full thirty-minute cardio workout before your weight-training session.

Similarly, you should always follow your workout with a cool-down period that consists of about five minutes of static stretching. Static stretching is discussed in the following section. Never statically stretch before engaging in any physical activity. Stretching a "cold" muscle increases the risk of injury and can hinder performance.

Your Workout Schedule

Your goal should be to fit working out into your lifestyle—make it part of your normal routine. As I mentioned in the previous section, I recommend doing your cardiovascular workout for thirty minutes three times a week. I also recommend doing your weight training workout three times a week. You have several options for accomplishing both of these goals.

(1) Do a thirty-minute cardio workout, followed by your weight training workout and static stretching, three times a week.

(2) Alternate your cardio and weight-training workouts. For example, do your thirty-minute cardio workout on Monday, Wednesday and Friday, and your weight-training workout on Tuesday, Thursday and Saturday. You can organize your schedule any way you like, but just make sure you don't do your total body weight-training workout two days in a row. As noted earlier, you need at least a twenty-four hour rest period between weight-training workouts. Keep in mind, it's okay to do your cardio workout two days in a row. If you do only a cardio workout, you should stretch at least your lower back and legs when you're done. If you use the arms on an elliptical, you should go through your entire stretching routine. (Stretching is discussed in Section V.)

(3) If you can devote only about thirty minutes, three days a week, to working out, you don't have to choose between your cardio workout and your weight-training workout. You can combine your cardio and weight-training workouts into one session (see "Cardio/Weight Training Combos" in Chapter Twelve). This combo workout will usually take between thirty and forty-five minutes.

(4) Finding time in your busy schedule for any exercising at all can be a challenge. For those who have not been able to start or stick to a regular exercise regimen due to time constraints, I've developed a concept called the "stretched out workout week" or SOWW. SOWW gives you nine days to fit in three total body weight training workouts and three or four cardio workouts. You can customize your workout schedule to accommodate changes in your daily, weekly or monthly routines. SOWW allows for unexpected events that interfere with your plans to work out on a given day. You can rest for two or even three days whenever it's necessary. But to achieve the full benefits of your weight-training workouts, try not to rest for more than three days on a regular basis. With SOWW, as long as you do three total body weight-

training workouts and three cardio workouts in nine days, you're adhering to a consistent exercise regimen.

The goal is to develop a realistic schedule that you can stick to. Consistency is essential. However, don't let that word, consistency, put pressure on you. Sometimes when people miss a few workouts in a row, they start to feel guilty. To avoid this pressure and guilt, they abandon their exercise regimens or avoid starting one in the first place. You need to be flexible and allow yourself to occasionally skip a workout or two. Then resume your regular schedule as soon as you can. Never exercise more intensely for a longer period of time during your next workout to make up for a missed one. This practice is not only unproductive, it can be dangerous.

If you're not feeling well, it's probably advisable to stop working out until you're feeling 100% again. Your body needs rest to recuperate from an illness. I would suggest asking your doctor whether you should stop exercising during an illness and when you can resume your workouts. The same is true for an injury.

One final suggestion: you may want to take a week off from working out every four to eight weeks. It's a good way to give your joints a rest.

Unlike caffeinated beverages and energy drinks, exercising is a healthy and natural way to boost your energy level. If you work out on a regular basis and have a sensible eating lifestyle, you'll find you have more energy all the time. Exercising may even improve your mood.

Important Medical Considerations

Have you heard this joke:

Patient: "Doctor, it hurts when I do this."

Doctor: "Then don't do that."

You should STOP exercising if you experience pain and consult your doctor. Even if the pain subsides or goes away, don't continue with your workout. Pain is your body's way of alerting you that an injury is imminent or has already occurred. Don't try to work through the pain or you may sustain or exacerbate an injury. Instead of "No pain. No gain," your motto should be "No pain. No pain."

Here's another old joke:

Doctor: "Have you had this pain before?"

Patient: "Yes."

Doctor: "Well you've got it again."

Recurring pain is often the reason people stop exercising, playing a sport, or engaging in their favorite physical activities. If recurring pain is preventing you from working toward your fitness goals, see your doctor so you can get treated for the condition that's causing the recurring pain.

While pain is not normal, soreness is, particularly for beginners. You may feel sore immediately after, or a day or two after, any strenuous physical activity. Initial soreness is common and should resolve itself in subsequent workouts. However, if the soreness gets worse, see your doctor. Warming up aerobically before working out and stretching afterward can limit or prevent soreness.

Pain is not the only reason to stop exercising. As noted in the previous section, if you feel nauseous, light-headed or dizzy, immediately STOP your workout and seek medical attention.

Chapter Eleven

Hustle, Hustle, Move Every Muscle: The Exercises

In this chapter, you'll find step-by-step instructions for performing exercises using weight-training machines. (After you thoroughly familiarize yourself with these instructions, you can consult the quick reference charts in Appendix Three for a handy reminder.) I've included exercises for a total body workout. You'll be working the muscles or muscle groups in the chest, back, shoulders, arms, legs and abdomen. I'll explain how to position yourself correctly to start the exercise and how to perform the exercise. Illustrations depicting the starting and ending positions accompany each exercise. You'll notice all of the exercises have two movements—a positive rep and a negative rep—except for the seated row, which has four movements. The written descriptions reflect traditional movement patterns for positive and negative reps. When you get to Chapter Twelve, you'll see how you can alter the traditional movement patterns to increase the intensity of the exercises.

CHEST

The pectoralis major and minor muscles in the chest are commonly referred to as the "pecs." To fully develop your chest muscles, you have to do two exercises:

- Bench Press
- Butterfly (Fly)

Vertical Bench Press on a Vertical Bench Press Machine

Getting Ready

(1) Sit down with your hips back in the seat so they form a 90 degree angle with your back.

(2) Adjust the seat up or down so that the bench press bar is at your chest height.

(3) Adjust the bar forward or back so that you can go through a full ROM without straining your shoulders to get your hands behind and on the hand grips.

(4) Grasp the horizontal handles with a palms-down grip. Your wrists should stay in the neutral position.

(5) Your elbows should be behind you and bent at about 90 degrees. Don't "flap" them.

(6) Your forearms should be about parallel to the floor.

(7) Keep your feet flat on the floor for stability.

(8) Don't shrug or raise your shoulders; relax them.

The Movement

(1) Push the bar away from you until there's a slight bend in your elbows. Don't lock out.

(2) Control the weight as you allow the bar to come back toward you. Stop before the weight plates touch to avoid resting.

(See Figure 1)

* Note: If your wrists are not in the neutral position but are hyper-extended (the back of your hands face you), you're placing stress on your wrist joints.

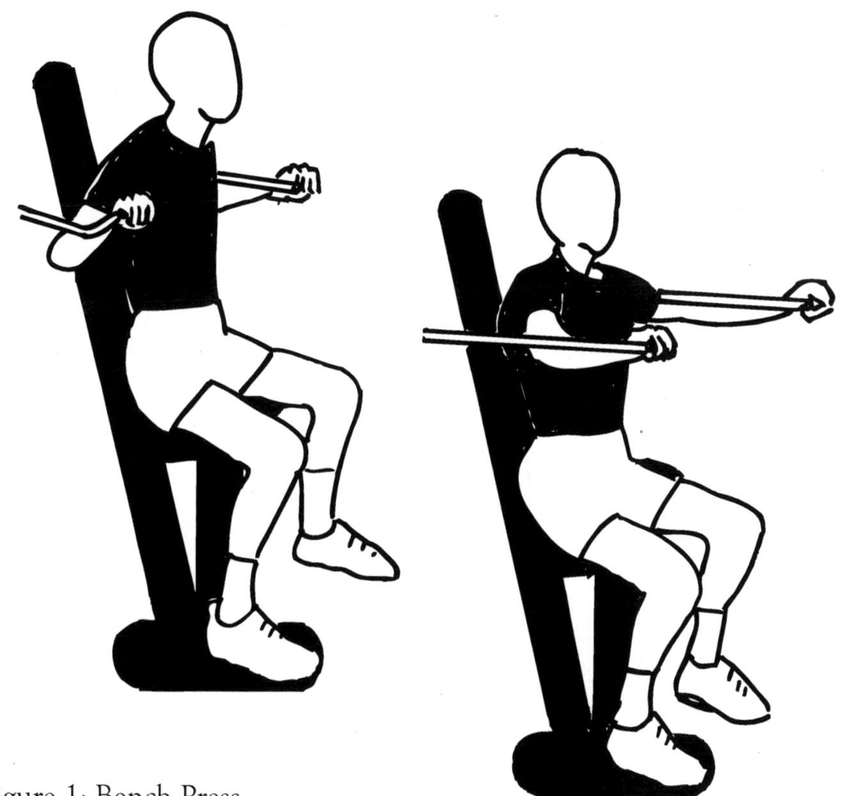

Figure 1: Bench Press

Vertical Butterfly (Fly) on a Pec Dec Machine

Getting Ready

(1) Move your hips back in the pec dec seat to ensure your back is supported.

(2) Adjust the seat up or down.

(3) Adjust the pec dec arms forward or back to ensure a full ROM.

(4) Place your forearms behind the arm pads.

(5) Your elbows should be bent at close to 90 degree angles.

(6) Grasp the round horizontal bars above the pads if the machine has them.

(7) Don't shrug or raise your shoulders; relax them.

The Movement

(1) Squeeze the pads together in front of your chest. Stop just before the pads touch each other.

(2) Allow your arms to move back to the starting position with a slow and controlled negative rep.

(See Figure 2)

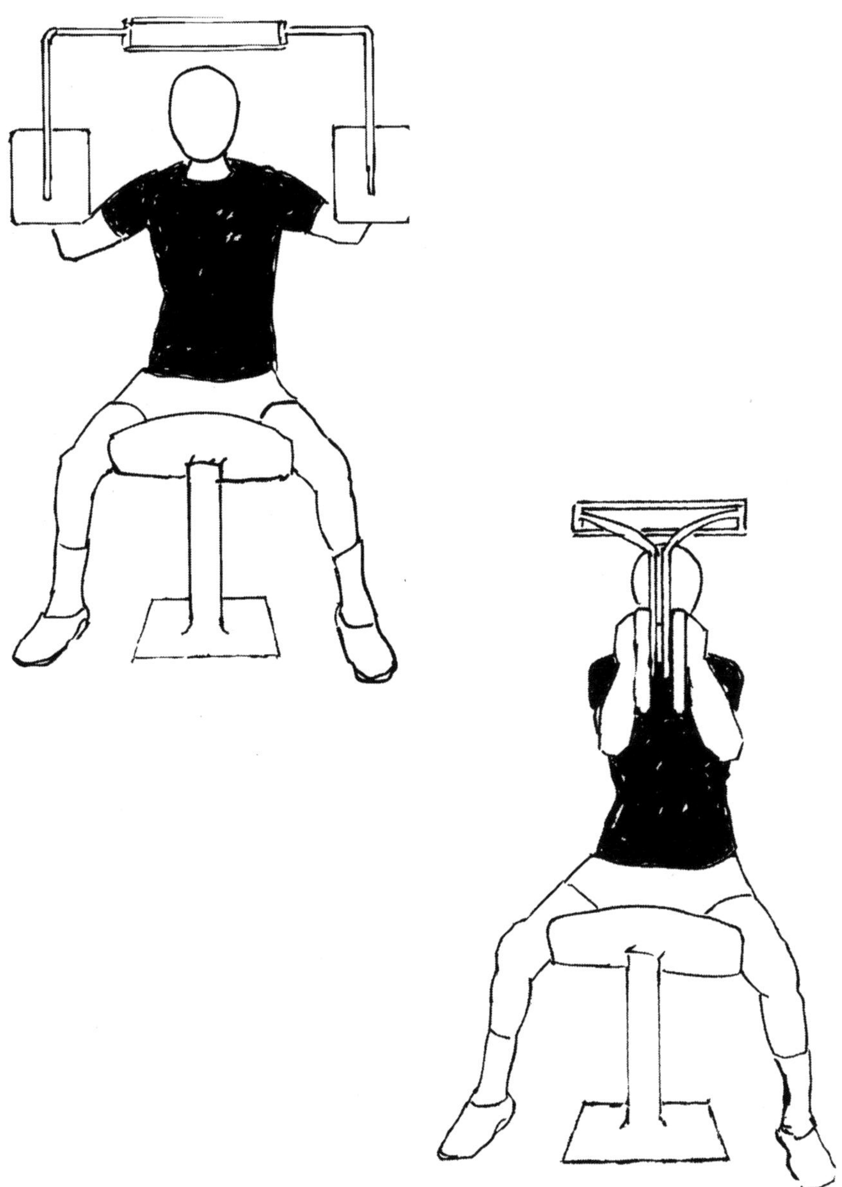

Figure 2: Vertical Butterfly

BACK (upper and lower)

The four-part seated row works both the large muscles in the upper back, called the latissimus dorsi or "lats," and the smaller muscles in the lower back, called the erector spinae or "erectors." You can do seated rows on a low row machine that has a footplate to prevent you from sliding forward, ensuring a full ROM. If space allows, you can also do seated rows on the floor using the lower pulley of a multi-station machine. You'll need to dig your heels into the floor to prevent sliding forward.

Four-part Seated Row

Getting Ready

(1) Attach a row handle (i.e., "double D" handle) to the cable of the low row machine or to the lower pulley of a multi-station machine.

(2) Sit on the bench with your legs fully extended (but not locked out), and place your feet on the footplate.

(3) Keep your feet firmly planted as you do the exercise.

(4) Grasp the row handle with your palms facing each other.

(5) Lean in, bending from the waist, and grasp the row handle. If there is slack in the cable or you're not feeling a stretch in your lower back, shimmy backward while holding the row handle until there is no slack in the cable and you feel the stretch.

The Movement

(1) Keeping your arms extended (don't pull the row handle toward you), sit back so that your back and hips form a 90 degree angle. Going beyond a 90 degree angle puts your lower back in an unsupported and vulnerable position. This first movement is the positive rep of the exercise for the lower back muscles.

(2) Pull the row handle toward your abdomen. Keep your elbows close

to your sides (don't flare them out). This second movement is the positive rep for the upper back muscles. Keep your back straight; don't lean back beyond 90 degrees to help pull the row handle into your abdomen. That's cheating.

(3) Control the weight as you extend your arms (straighten them). Maintain the 90 degree angle with your back and hips. The third movement is the negative rep for the upper back muscles.

(4) Control the weight and lean in from your waist to the starting position. You should again feel a stretch in your lower back. This fourth movement is the negative rep for the lower back muscles and brings you back to the starting position.

(See Figure 3)

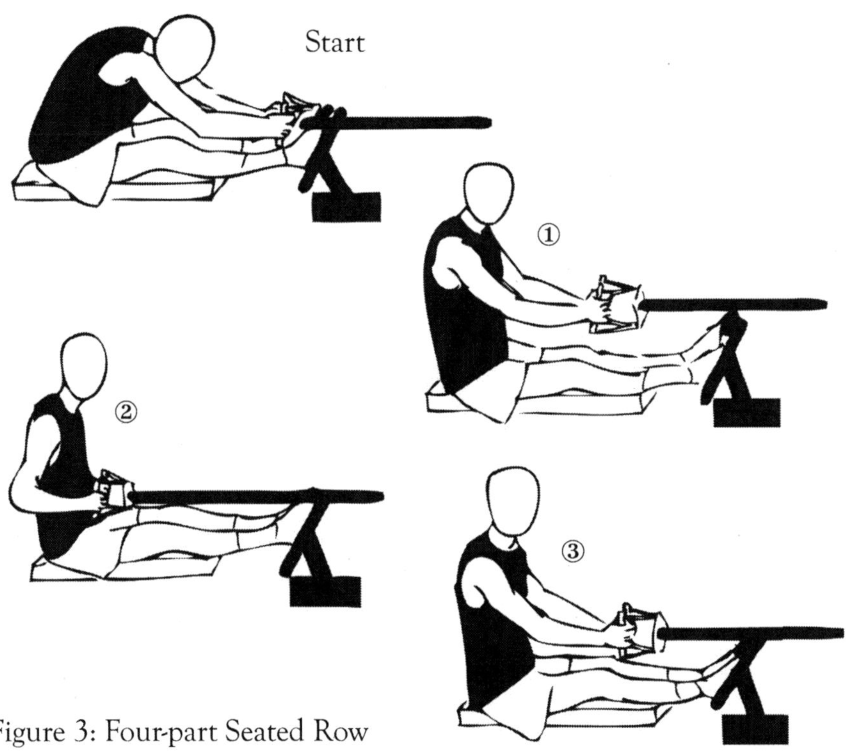

Figure 3: Four-part Seated Row

SHOULDERS

The shoulder press works the shoulder muscle (deltoid or "delts").

Shoulder Press

Getting Ready

(1) Sit down in the seat of the shoulder press machine with your hips all the way back to form a 90 degree angle with your back.
(2) Grasp the horizontal handles of the shoulder press bar with your palms facing out (away from you) and your wrists in the neutral position.
(3) Adjust the seat height so that your elbows are bent at about 45 degree angles, and the handles are at shoulder height.
(4) Don't shrug your shoulders; relax them.

The Movement

(1) Press the bar upward until just before lock-out. Keep your wrists in the neutral position.
(2) Control the bar as you allow it to come down to a point just before the weight plates touch.

(See Figure 4)

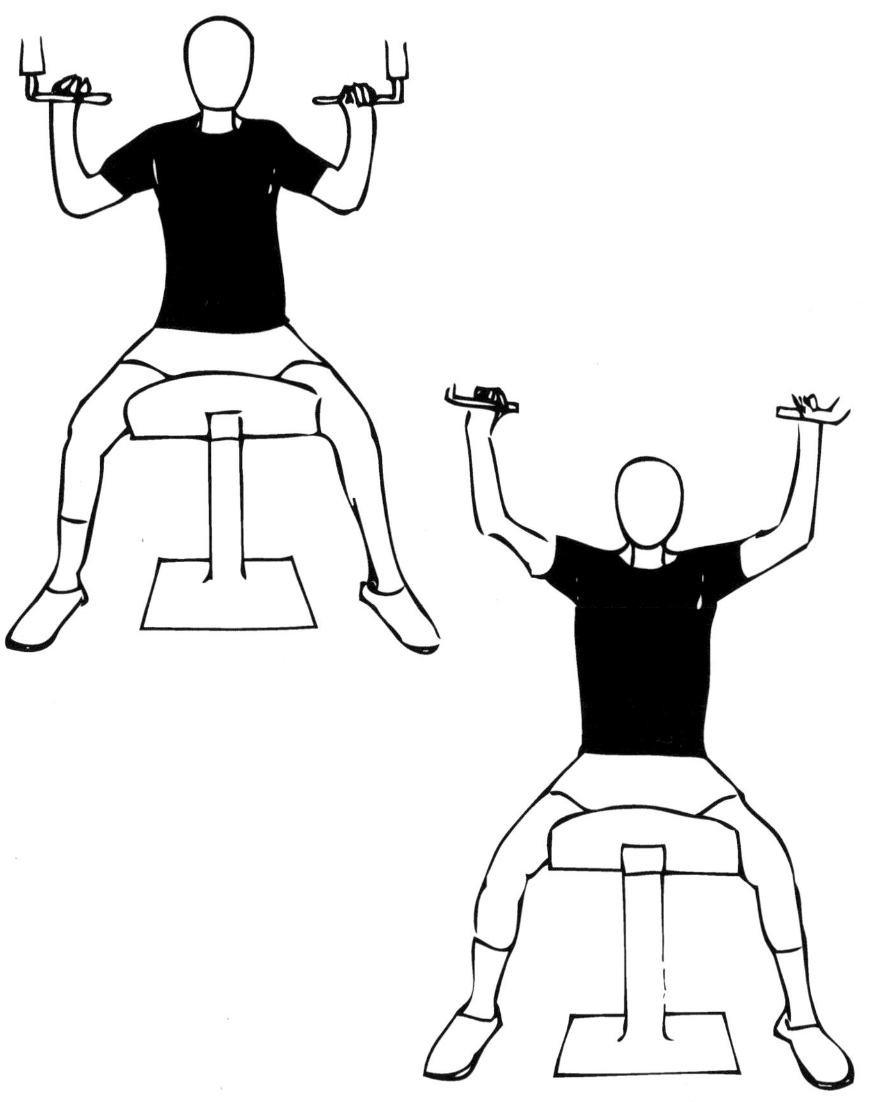

Figure 4: Shoulder Press

ARMS

To fully develop your arms, you have to do three exercises:

- Triceps press-downs OR triceps extensions for the triceps muscles in the back of the upper arms (using an upper pulley).
- Biceps curls for the biceps muscles in the front of the upper arms (using a lower pulley).
- Wrist curls for the muscles in the bottom of the forearms (using a lower pulley).
- Reverse wrist curls for the muscles in the top of the forearms (using a lower pulley).

Triceps Press-downs

Getting Ready

(1) Attach a short straight bar, lat bar (a long bar with downward angled hand grips), or accessory piece (e.g., rope handles or inverted "V" bar) to an upper pulley cable.

(2) Stand facing the weight plates.

(3) Grasp the bar with a palms down grip and your hands either shoulder width apart or thumbs width apart (i.e., both thumbs extend out along the bar until the tips touch).

(4) Bring the bar down until your elbows are bent at about 45 degree angles.

(5) Keep your elbows at your sides and your wrists in neutral position throughout every repetition.

The Movement

(1) Push (press) the bar down toward your thighs by straightening (extending) your arms. Don't lock out.

(2) Control the bar as it comes back to the starting position, with your elbows bent at about 45 degree angles.

(See Figure 5)

* Note: Remember to keep your elbows against your sides and your wrists in neural position throughout every repetition.

* Note: A lat bar is heavier than a short straight bar. Rope handles and the inverted V bar make it harder to do triceps press-downs. You may have to lift lighter weight when you use each of these accessories.

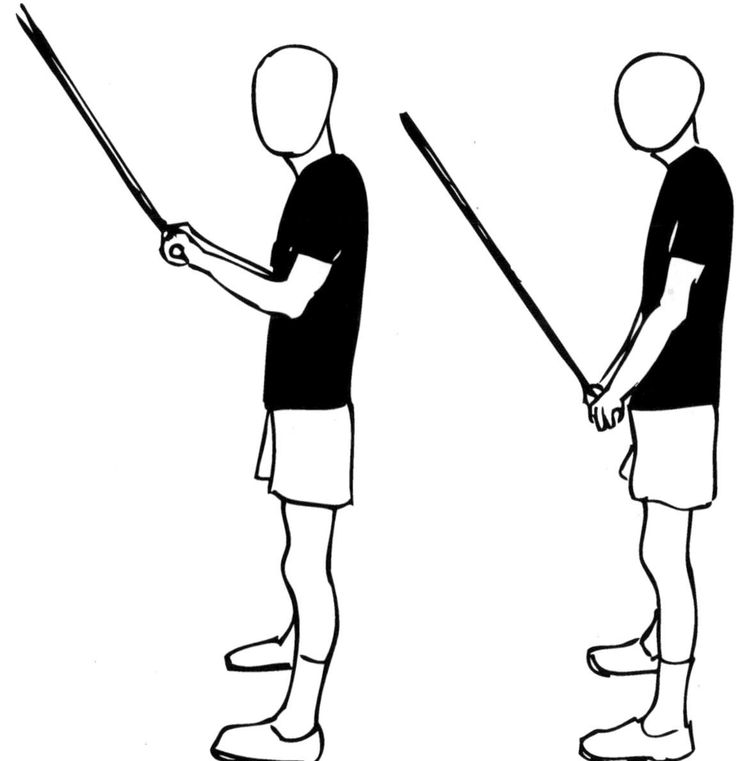

Figure 5: Triceps Press-downs

Triceps Extensions

Getting Ready

(1) Attach a short straight bar or lat bar (a long bar with downward angled hand grips) to an upper pulley cable.

(2) Stand facing the weight plates.

(3) Grasp the bar with a palms up grip and your hands shoulder width apart.

(4) Bring the bar down until your elbows are bent at about 45 degree angles.

(5) Keep your elbows against your sides and your wrists in neutral position throughout every repetition.

The Movement

(1) Pull the bar down toward your thighs by straightening (extending) your arms. Don't lock out.

(2) Control the bar as it returns to the starting position, with your elbows bent at about 45 degree angles.

(See Figure 6)

* Note: Remember to keep your elbows against your sides and your wrists in neutral position throughout every repetition.

* Note: A lat bar is heavier than a short straight bar. You may have to lift lighter weight when you use the lat bar.

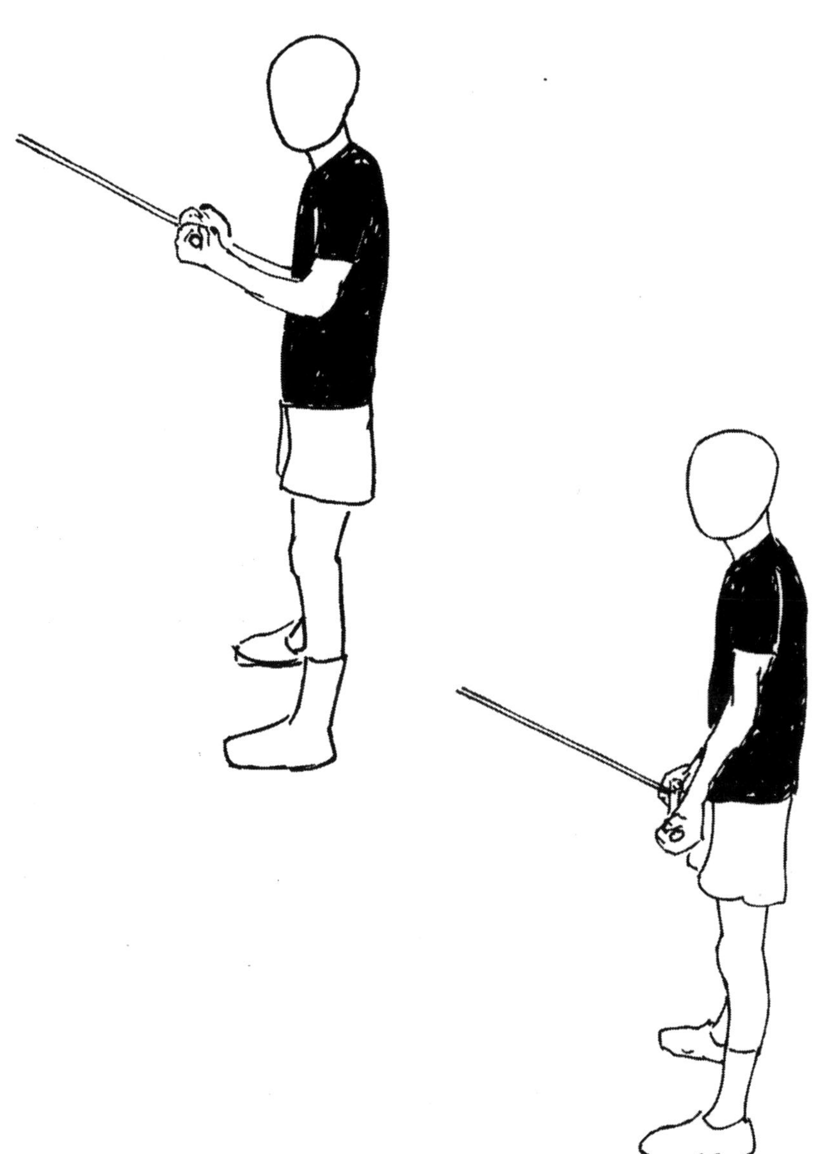

Figure 6: Triceps Extensions

Two Arm Biceps Curls

Getting Ready

(1) Attach a short straight bar or "easy curl" bar to a lower pulley cable.

(2) Stand facing the weight plates.

(3) Grasp the bar with a palms up grip and your hands shoulder width apart. (Grasp the easy curl bar on the angled areas.)

(4) Your arms should be fully extended (but not locked out) down in front of you.

(5) Keep your elbows against your sides and your wrists in neutral position throughout every repetition.

The Movement

(1) Bend (flex) your arms at the elbows to curl the bar up toward your chest. Don't bend your elbows as much as you can physically bend them to avoid resting the muscles.

(2) Control the bar as you return to the starting position, with a slight bend in your elbows.

(See Figure 7)

* Note: Remember to keep your elbows against your sides and your wrists in neutral position throughout every repetition. If you flex (bend) your wrists on the positive reps, your forearm flexor muscles will be helping the biceps curl the weight.

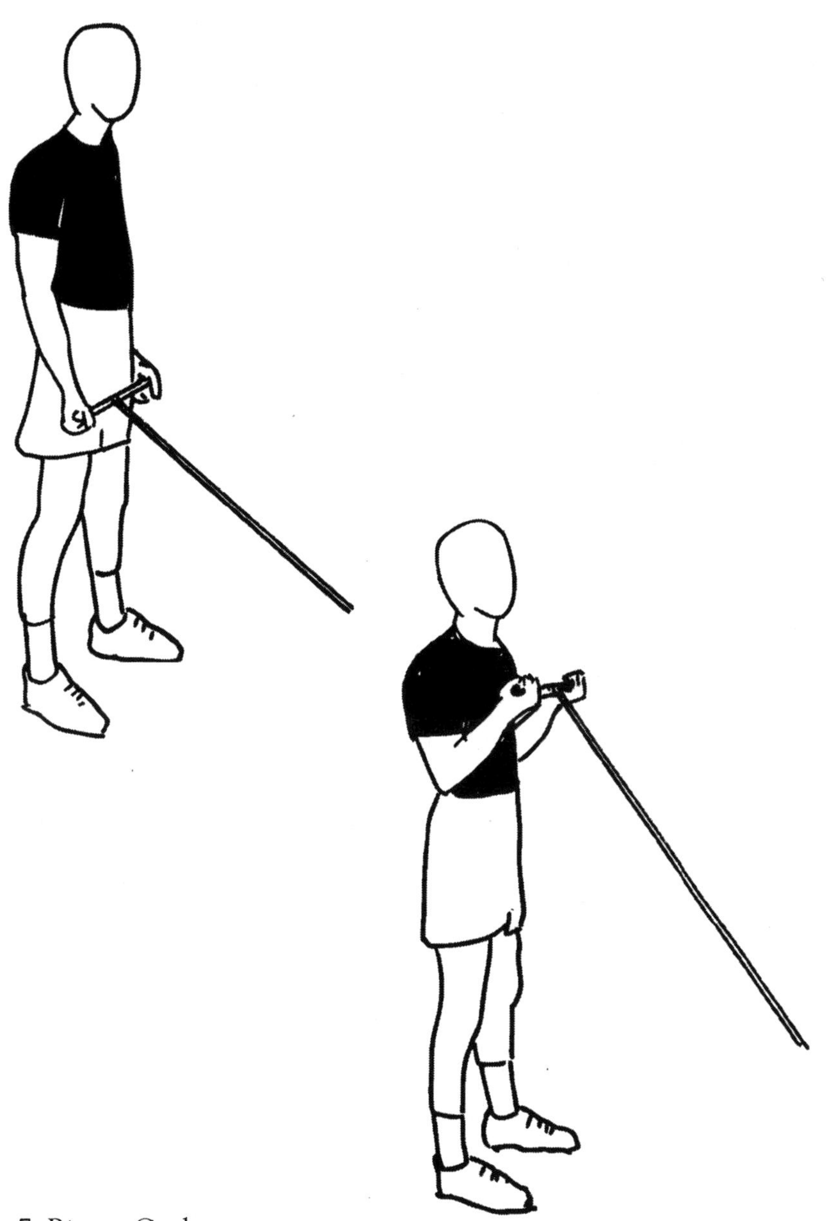

Figure 7: Biceps Curls

Wrist Curls

Getting Ready

(1) Attach a short straight bar to a lower pulley cable.

(2) Stand facing the weight plates with your arms fully extended (but not locked out) down in front of you.

(3) Grasp the bar with a palms up grip and your hands shoulder width apart.

The Movement

(1) Use the same curling movement as in the biceps curl, but instead of bending your elbows, bend (flex) your wrists.

(2) Control the bar as you return to the starting position, with a slight bend at your wrists.

(See Figure 8)

* Note: As a general rule, you can use at least as much weight, if not more, for wrist curls as you use for biceps curls.

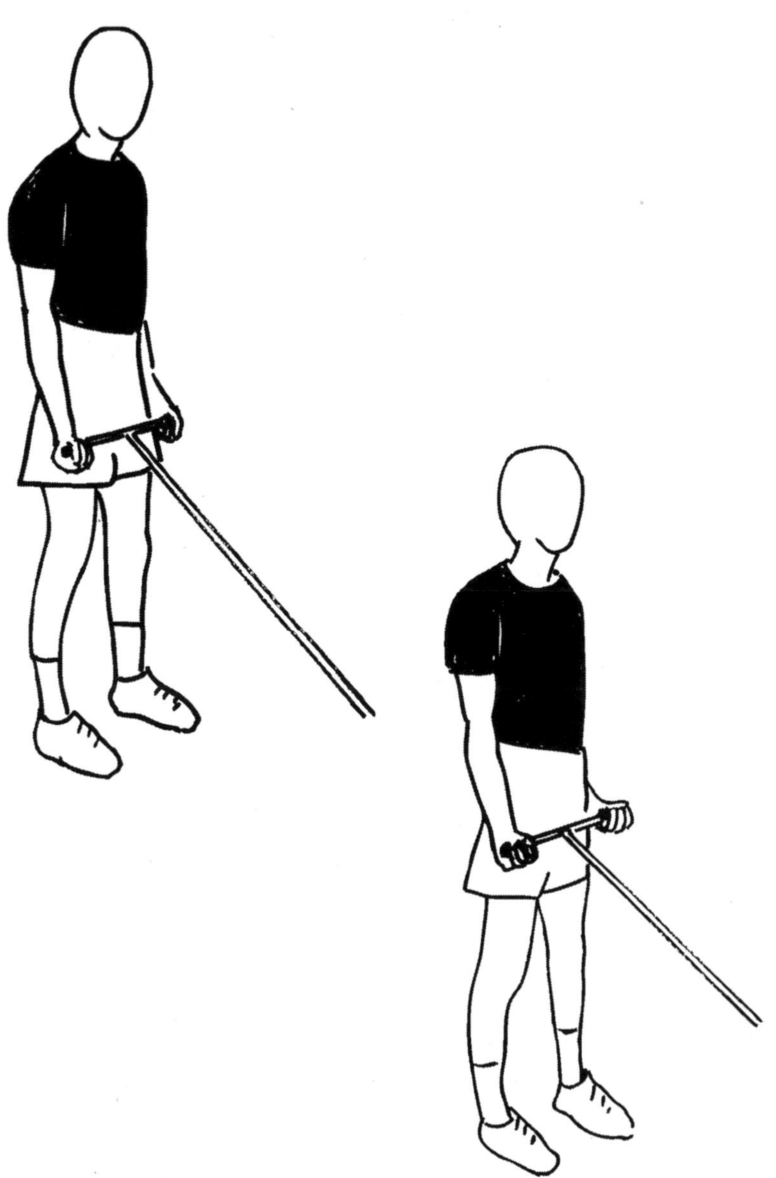

Figure 8: Wrist Curls

Reverse Wrist Curls

Getting Ready

(1) Use a short straight bar on a lower pulley cable.
(2) Stand facing the weight plates with your arms fully extended (but not locked out) down in front of you.
(3) Grasp the bar with a palms down grip and your hands shoulder width apart.
(4) Your wrists should be in the neutral position.

The Movement

(1) Reverse curl your wrists (the backs of your hands curl up and face you) as you bend your arms at the elbow. At the end of the positive rep, your palms will be almost facing the ceiling.
(2) On the negative rep, un-curl your wrists as you straighten your arms to the starting position.

(See Figure 9)

* Note: In this exercise your elbows are moving. That's okay. Even though you're doing the biceps curl movement, you're isolating the forearm extensor muscles because you're using a palms down grip. When you do a biceps curl you use a palms up grip.

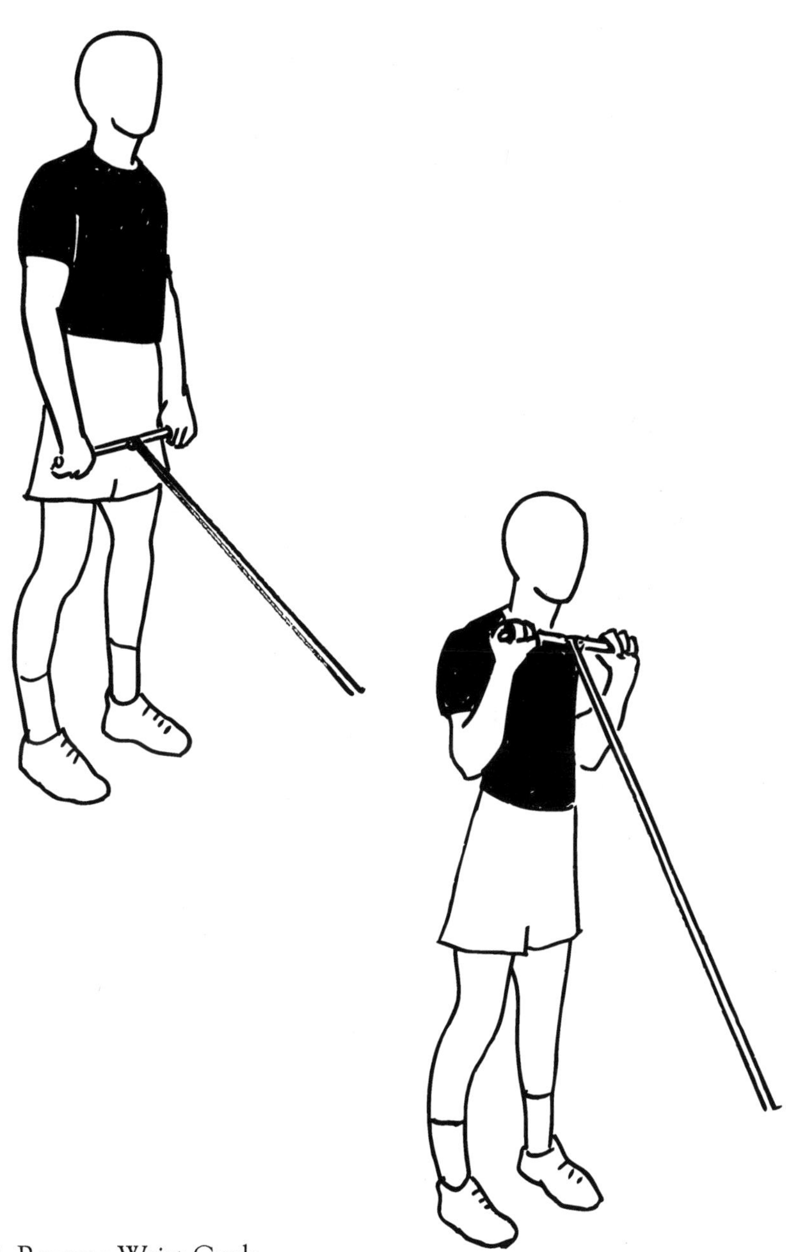

Figure 9: Reverse Wrist Curls

LEGS

I recommend four exercises for the leg muscles:

- Leg extensions for the quadriceps femoris or "quads," the muscles in the front of your thighs.
- Leg curls for your hamstrings or "hams," the muscles in the back of your thighs.
- Leg press for the quads, hams and "glutes,"the muscles that shape the buttocks.
- Calf raises for the gastrocnemius or "gastroc," the muscles in the back of your lower legs.

An additional exercise is optional:

- Inner-outer thigh pulls for the adductor muscles (in the inner thighs) and abductor muscles (in the outer thighs). I suggest that you do inner-outer thigh pulls only if you engage in the following activities: skiing, ice skating, roller skating, roller blading and horseback riding.

Leg Extensions

Getting Ready

(1) Adjust the seat (forward or back) and padded bar to accommodate your height and leg length.

(2) Sit down and place your feet behind and under the lower padded bar. Your legs should be bent at the knees at a bit less than a 90 degree angle so you can go through a full ROM.

(3) Make sure the backs of your knees are in contact with the front edge of the seat. If you leave a space, your knee joints will be vulnerable to pressure and strain, increasing the risk of injury.

The Movement

(1) Lift the padded bar by extending (straightening) your legs to a point just before your knees lock out.

(2) Control the padded bar as it comes down to a point just before the weight plates touch.

(See Figure 10)

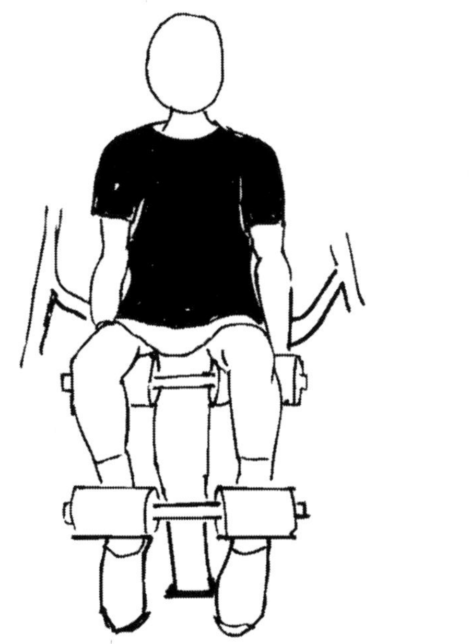

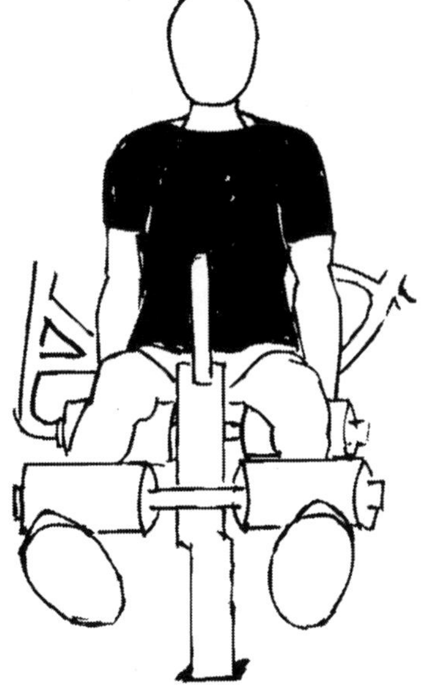

Figure 10: Leg Extensions

Leg Curls

Getting Ready

(1) Adjust the seat (forward or back) and the padded bar in front of the leg curl machine to accommodate your height and leg length.

(2) Sit in the seat of the leg curl machine.

(3) Extend your legs and put your heels on top of the padded bar.

(4) Move the padded bar above your knees down until it touches your legs above the kneecaps. The bar keeps your upper legs planted on the seat. It should never press down on your kneecaps when doing leg curls.

The Movement

(1) Curl the padded bar down and back as far as the machine will allow. A full ROM will usually allow your heels to end up slightly under the front edge of the seat.

(2) Control the weight as the bar comes up and stop just before the weight plates touch.

(See Figure 11)

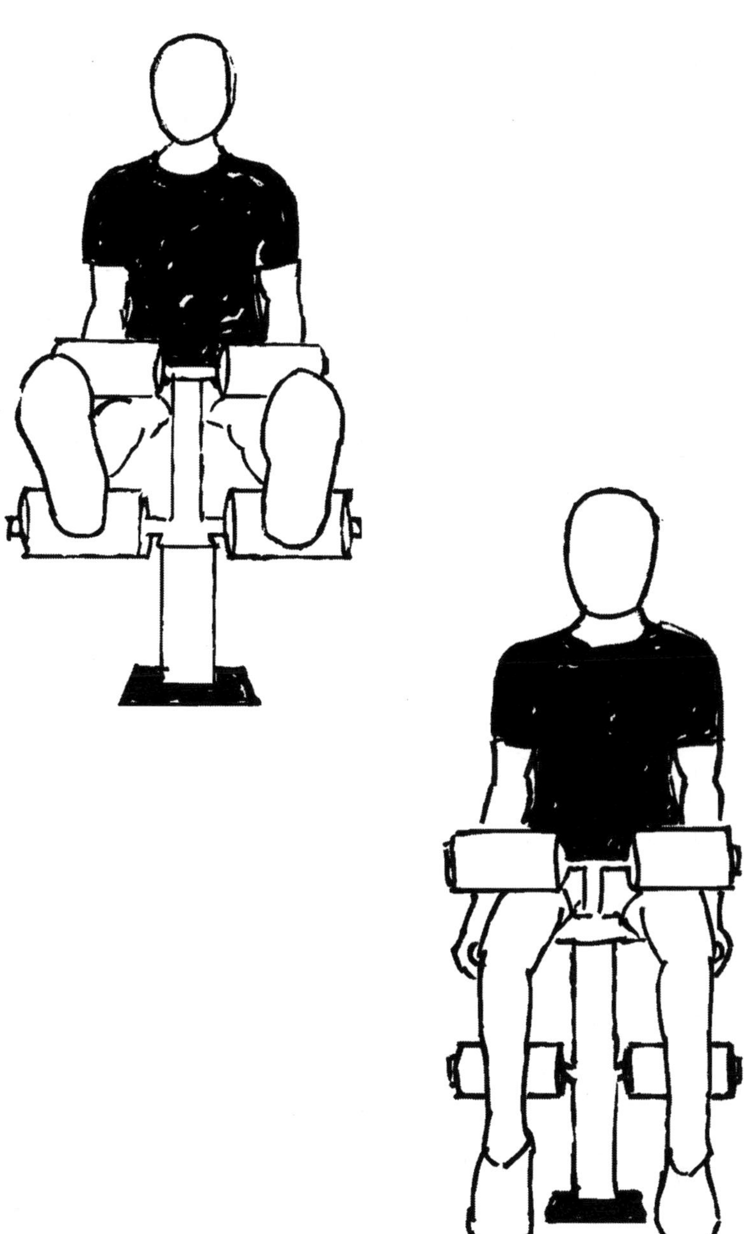

Figure 11: Leg Curls

Leg Press

Getting Ready

(1) Sit in the seat of the leg press machine with your back against the back support.

(2) Place your feet about shoulder width apart on the footplate (in the middle).

(3) Extend your legs a bit and push the footplate up so that you can unlock it. Move the handles on either side of you with your hands to unlock the footplate.

(4) Once unlocked, the footplate will move freely up and down. When you're done, lock the footplate.

The Movement

(1) Push the footplate up by extending (straightening) your legs to a point just before your knees lock out.

(2) Control the footplate as it comes down to a point just before rest, with your knees near your chest.

(See Figure 12)

* Note: If you have a home gym with a leg press attachment, you will be sitting upright. The attachment is parallel to the floor. On most leg press units the seat is adjustable back and forth and the footplate moves. On some machines the footplate is fixed and you move backward in the seat.

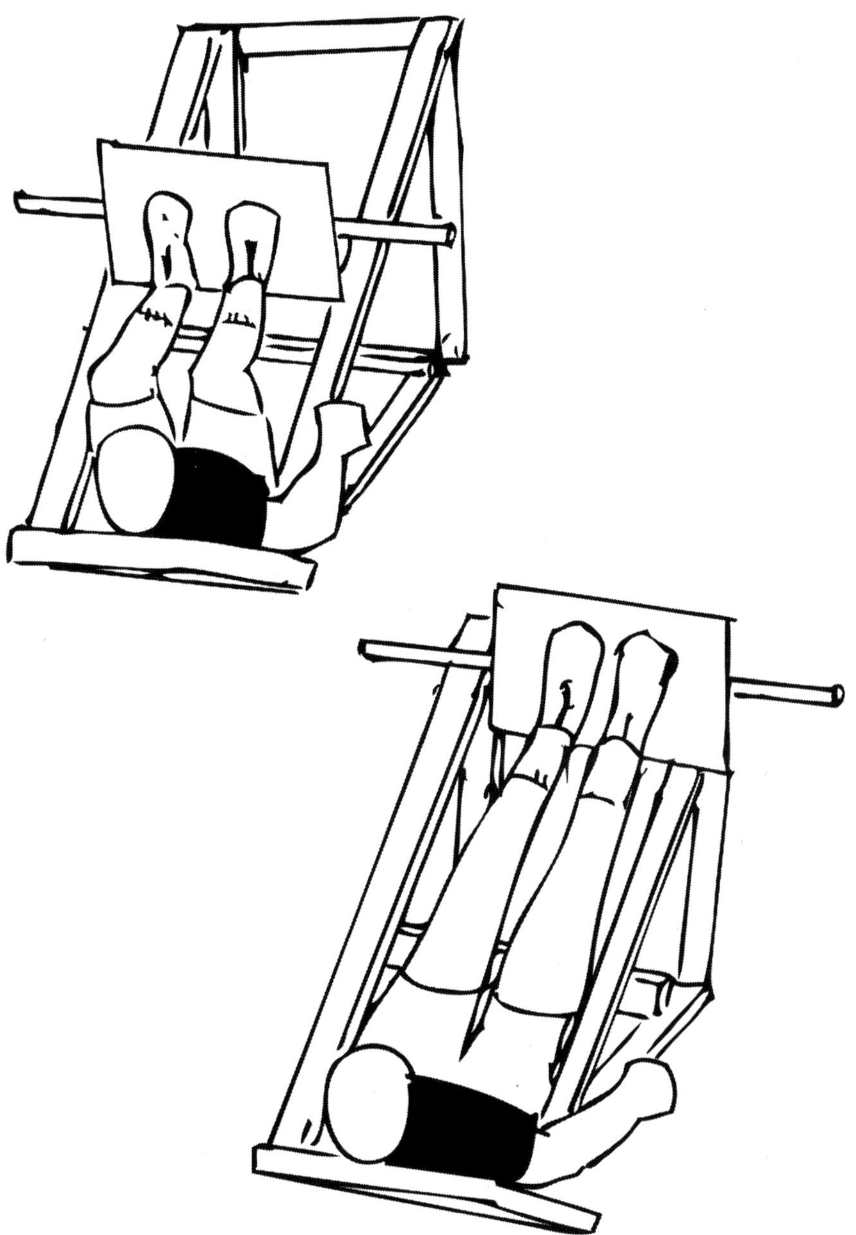

Figure 12: Leg Press

Calf Raises

Getting Ready

(1) After you complete the leg presses, you have to change the position of your feet on the footplate to do calf raises. Extend your legs and move the footplate up. Hold it up while you move your feet down to the lower part of the footplate, so that only the balls of your feet and toes are on it.

(2) Your feet should be fully flexed so that your heels will be under and slightly in front of the bottom edge of the footplate. If you don't feel secure moving your feet while the footplate is unlocked, lock it, move your feet down, and unlock it.

The Movement

(1) With your legs extended, but not locked out, push the footplate away from you as if you were standing on your toes.

(2) On the negative rep, allow your heels to go under and in front of the footplate (the starting position). You should feel a stretch in your calf muscles.

(See Figure 13)

* Note: You can also work your calf muscles on a free-standing (FSU) unit with a fixed footplate. The movements are the same as on the leg press machine, but when you straighten your legs, you move instead of the footplate.

(See Figure 14)

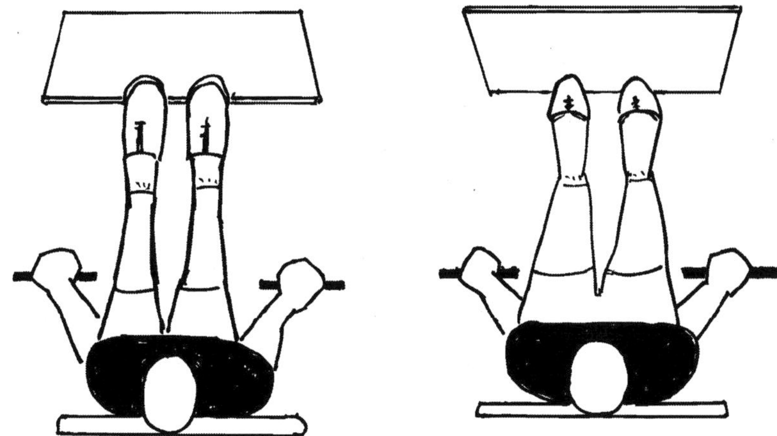

Figure 13: Calf Raises

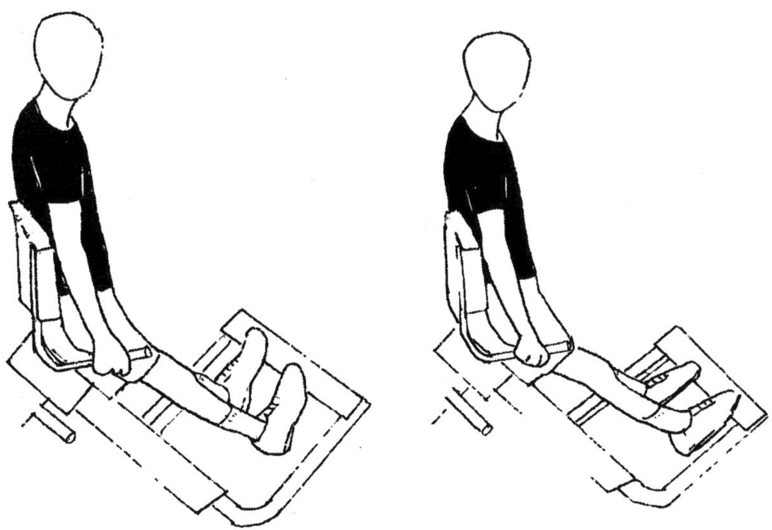

Figure 14: Calf Raises on a Free-standing Unit

Inner-Outer Thigh Pulls

Getting Ready

(1) Sit in the seat of the adductor-abductor machine and place your legs in the "L" shaped padded brackets.

   (a) To work the adductors (inner thigh muscles), spread your legs and place the vertical parts of the "L" brackets against the insides of your legs.

   (b) To work the abductors (outer thigh muscles), keep your legs together and place the vertical parts of the "L" brackets against the outsides of your legs.

(2) Place your feet in the foot rests.

(3) Adjust the foot rests to ensure a full ROM in both directions.

(4) Grasp the handles on the sides of the seat for support.

(5) Do one set of inner thigh pulls then one set of outer thigh pulls or vice versa.

The Movement

(1) To work the adductors, bring your legs together. To work the abductors, spread your legs apart.

(2) Control the weight as you return to the starting position for each exercise.

(See Figure 15)

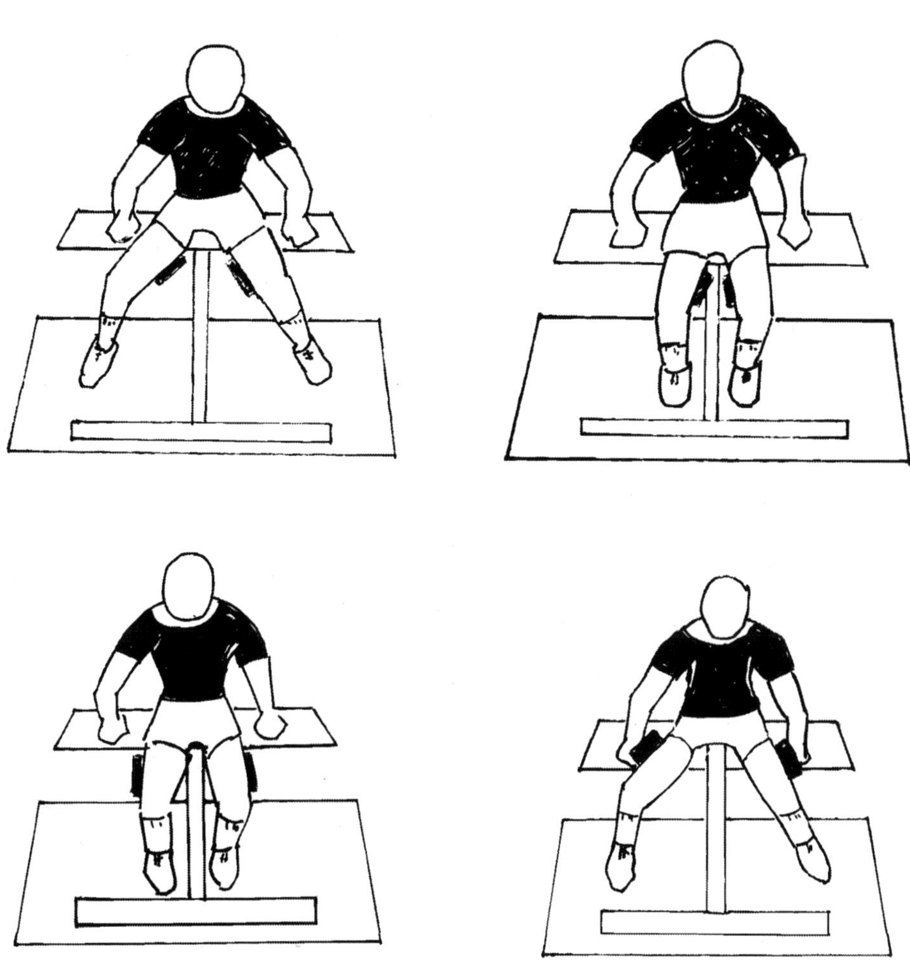

Figure 15: Inner Thigh Pulls (top), Outer Thigh Pulls (bottom)

ABDOMEN

You can work the three abdominal muscles–rectus abdominis (RA), internal obliques (IO) (sides), and external obliques (EO) (sides) on a mat, or on a machine and a free-standing unit. Many people spend too much time working their abs in their quest for a "six pack." But doing one set of an abdominal muscle exercise is just as effective as doing one set for any of the other exercises. You wouldn't spend thirty minutes a day working your triceps, quads or any other muscles. So why spend this much time on your abs? Spending too much time working your abs will not yield better or quicker results; it will only increase the potential for injuring your lower back. Keep in mind, you won't see any definition in your abdominal area, or anywhere else, unless you lower your body's percentage of excess fat and increase the percentage of lean body mass (muscle). As noted earlier, you accomplish this by adhering to a sensible eating lifestyle and a regular exercise regimen.

Crunches (Curl-ups) on a Mat

Getting Ready

(1) Lie on your back with your knees bent and feet flat on the mat.
(2) Clasp your hands behind your head.

The Movement

(1) Lift your chest, head and shoulders up off the mat. Look up at the ceiling to avoid tucking your chin into your chest. Don't come all the way up to your knees by bending at the waist. A curl-up has a limited range of motion. When you feel the contraction in the upper part of your abdomen you've completed the positive rep.
(2) Control your movement back down to the starting position.

(See Figure 16)

* Note: If you're flapping your arms to help you do the crunch, that's cheating. Try keeping your arms close to the sides of your head to avoid flapping them.

* Note: Curl-ups work the upper part of the RA muscle, which extends vertically up and down the front of the abdomen. Curl-ups also work the IO muscles, which extend from the outer edges of the RA out to the sides.

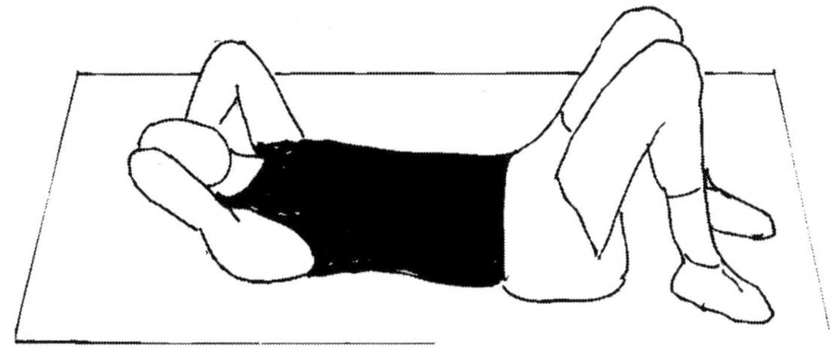

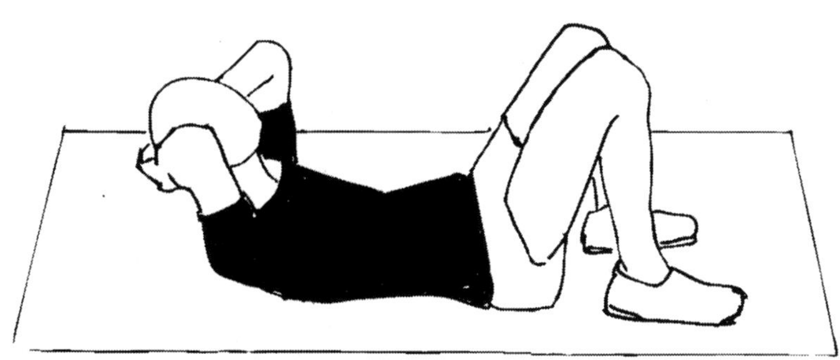

Figure 16: Crunches on a Mat

Reverse Crunches (Reverse Curl-ups) on a Mat

Getting Ready

(1) Lie on your back with your knees bent and your feet flat on the mat.

(2) Keep your arms fully extended at your sides.

(3) Place your hands palms down on the mat for stability.

The Movement

(1) Curl your knees toward your chest.

(2) Keep your legs bent and close together as you raise and lower them. Stop just before your feet touch the mat.

(See Figure 17)

* Note: Don't bounce or push off the mat. That's cheating. And don't rest your feet on the mat between reps; keep the contractions going throughout every repetition.

* Note: Reverse crunches work the lower part of the RA. They also work the EO muscles, which extend from the outer edges of the RA out to the sides. They're above the IO muscles. Unlike curl-ups, you should feel the burn a bit lower down across your abdomen and out to the sides when you do the reverse curl-ups.

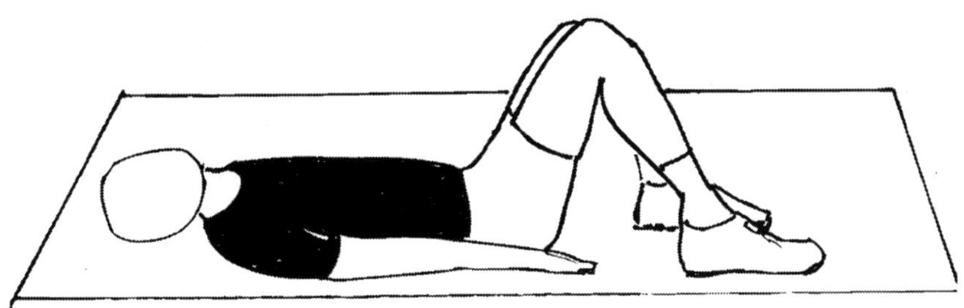

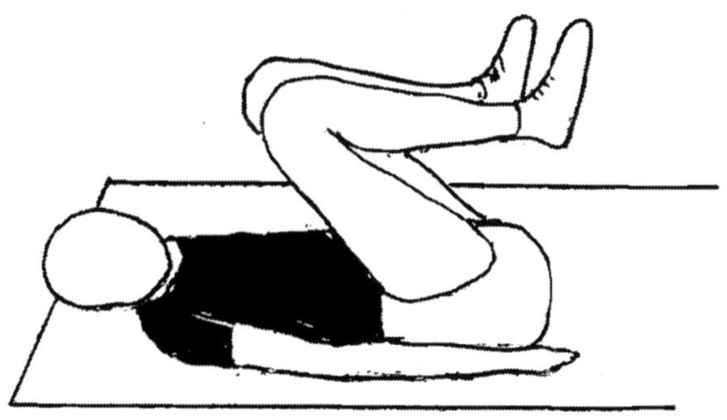

Figure 17: Reverse Crunches on a Mat

Combo Crunch on a Mat

Getting Ready

(1) Lie on your back with your knees bent and your feet flat on the mat.
(2) Clasp your hands behind your head.

The Movement

(1) Simultaneously do a curl-up and a reverse curl-up: bring your chest, head, shoulders and knees up together and down together.
(2) Slowly and smoothly lower your chest, head, shoulders and knees together.

(See Figure 18)

* Note: Don't flap your arms, tuck your chin into your chest, or bounce your feet off the mat.

* Note: Combo crunches work the upper and lower parts of the RA and the obliques simultaneously. But it may require practice to coordinate the two movements. Start with a low number of reps, and gradually increase.

* Note: I'm not recommending exercises designed specifically for the obliques in this book because they involve twisting, rotating and side bending movements, which can strain your lower back muscles, a common concern. Crunches, reverse crunches and combo crunches are adequate for working your obliques.

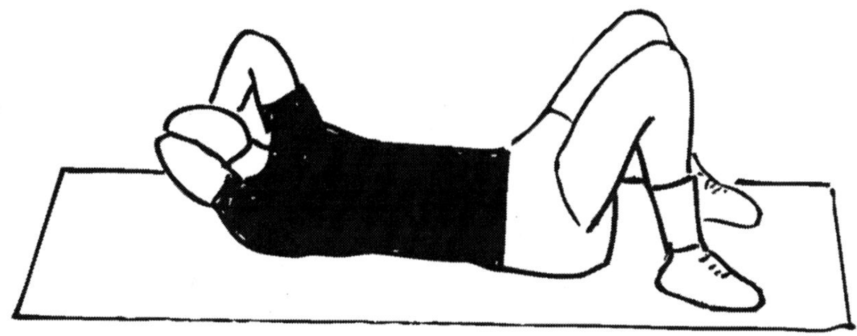

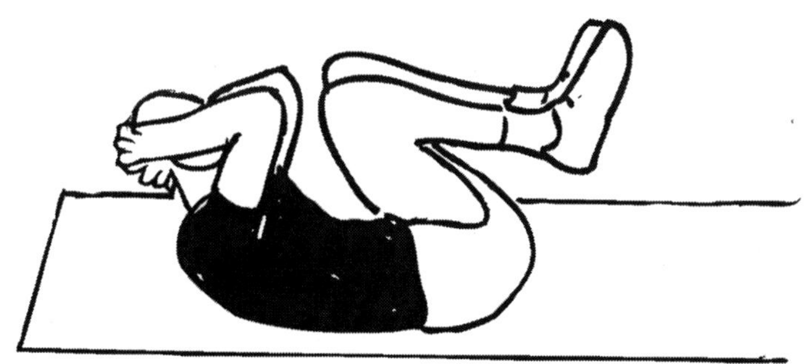

Figure 18: Combo Crunches on a Mat

Crunches on an Abdominal Crunch (Ab Crunch) Machine

Getting Ready

(1) Adjust the seat up or down so that you can keep your head on the head support pad, preventing you from bringing your chin toward your chest.

(2) Place your elbows on the pads.

(3) Grasp the vertical handles behind the pads.

(4) Place your feet behind the roller pads or padded bar.

The Movement

(1) Move your chest toward your thighs.

(2) Control the weight as you move back to a point just before the weight plates touch.

(See Figure 19)

* Note: If you feel any strain in your lower back or neck, stop. If the strain occurs whenever you use the machine, do curl-ups on a mat.

* Note: The ab crunch machine has its own weight stack. You can increase the intensity of the exercise by choosing a heavier weight.

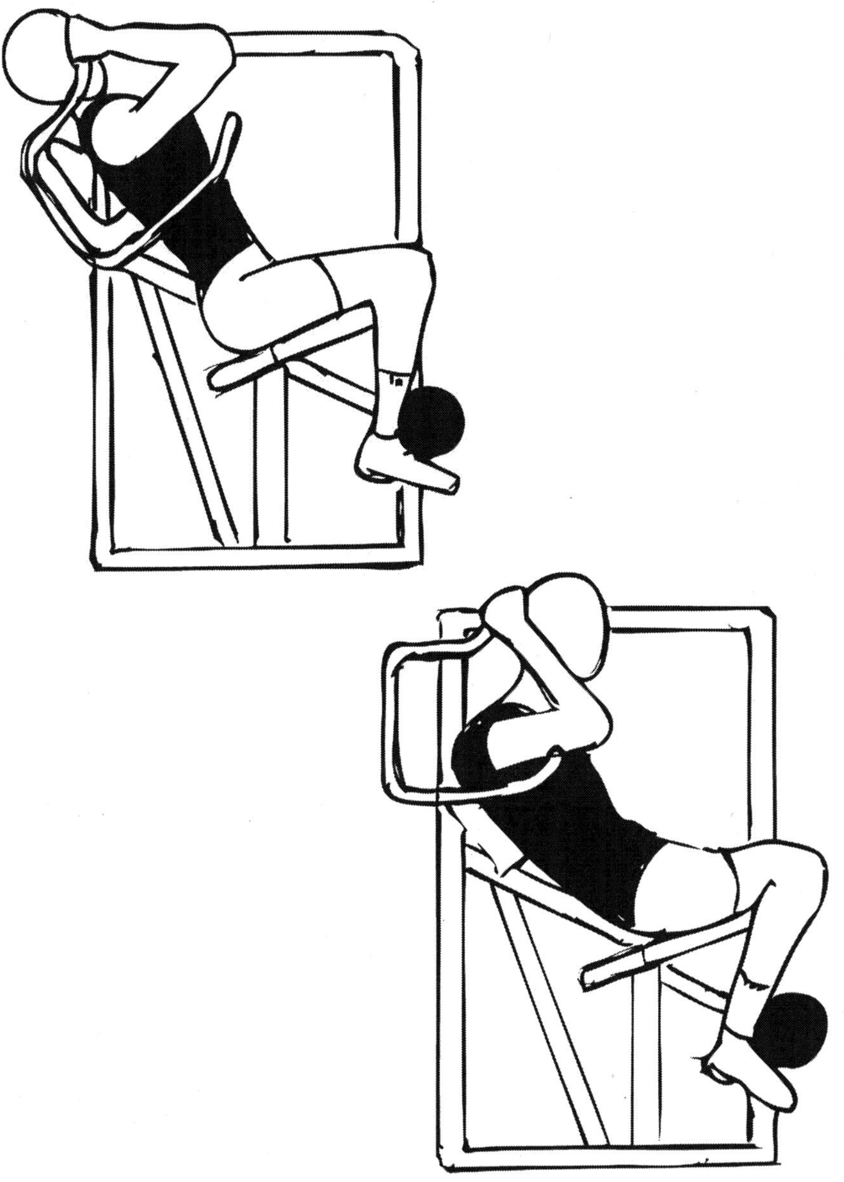

Figure 19: Crunches on an Ab Crunch Machine

Vertical Knee Raises on a Vertical Knee Raise (VKR) Free-standing Unit

Getting Ready

(1) Stand facing away from the unit but directly in front of the back support pad.

(2) Place your forearms on the horizontal arm pads.

(3) Grasp the vertical handles just in front of the pads.

(4) Step up onto the foot platforms.

(5) Press your back against the back pad, which has a slight backward angle.

(6) Take your feet off the foot platform and keep your legs together. They will be dangling.

The Movement

(1) Lift both knees up toward your chest. Keep your knees as close to your body as possible and your back against the back support pad.

(2) Slowly lower your knees to the starting position.

(See Figure 20)

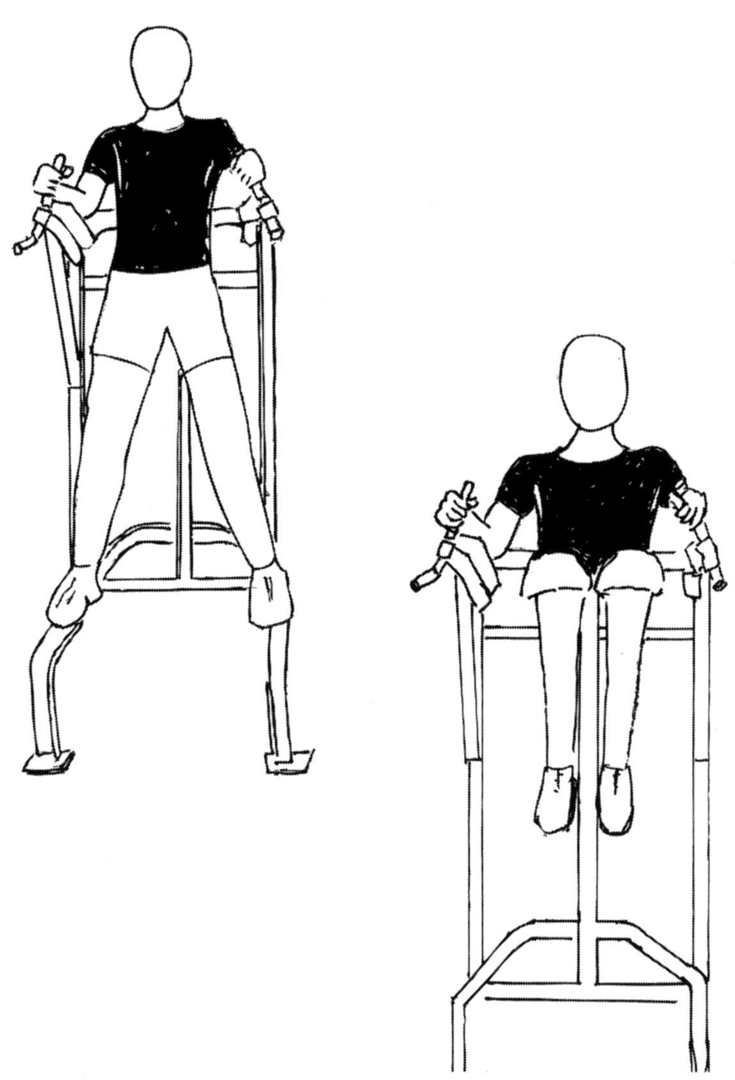

Figure 20: Vertical Knee Raises

Chapter Twelve

Putting It All Together: Your Workout Program

In Chapter Ten, we went over the basic information you need to build muscle strength and endurance through weight training. In Chapter Eleven, we discussed how to perform the exercises. Now you're ready to put it all together and begin your workout program.

As noted in Chapter Ten, you should warm up before every weight-training workout by doing an aerobic exercise for five to ten minutes. When you're ready to begin your weight-training session, it's generally recommended that you start with the largest muscles and work your way to the smallest. Following are the upper body muscles in order of largest to smallest: pecs (chest), lats (back), delts (shoulders), triceps, biceps, forearms. Following are the lower body muscles in order of largest to smallest: quads, hams, gastrocs. Ab exercises can be done at any point in a workout.

Following are two weight-training workout routines. I recommend you alternate between them. For your legs, the first routine includes the leg press, and the second includes leg extensions and leg curls. For your abs, the first routine includes crunches and reverse crunches, and the second includes combo crunches.

Workout Routine One

(1) Leg Press
(2) Bench Press
(3) Calf Raises
(4) Pec Dec
(5) Crunches
(6) Four-part Seated Row
(7) Reverse Crunches
(8) Shoulder Press
(9) Triceps Press-downs OR Triceps Extensions
(10) Biceps Curls
(11) Wrist Curls
(12) Reverse Wrist Curls

Workout Routine Two

(1) Leg Extensions
(2) Bench Press
(3) Leg Curls
(4) Pec Dec
(5) Calf Raises
(6) Four-part Seated Row
(7) Combo Crunches
(8) Shoulder Press
(9) Triceps Press-downs OR Triceps Extensions
(10) Biceps Curls
(11) Wrist Curls
(12) Reverse Wrist Curls

In both workout routines you're alternating between the largest upper body muscles and the largest lower body muscles. The routines are efficient and effective for nearly all individuals, from the beginner to the highly trained. Following are some options for changing the routines to keep your workouts interesting and to avoid wasting time if a machine you need is already in use:

- Start with an upper body exercise instead of a lower body exercise.
- Work your upper body large to small muscles then your lower body large to small muscles or vice versa.
- Do your leg presses and calf raises back to back on a leg press machine.
- Do an ab exercise in between an upper and lower body exercise.
- Do your abs last (before stretching).
- If a machine is in use, skip to the next largest muscle or do an ab exercise, then go back to the machine you skipped.

Suggested Workout Programs

I'm going to recommend four stand-alone workout programs and seven combination (combo) workout programs for you to choose from. You can do one workout for a few weeks, then switch to another, and continue to rotate through the options. Varying your workout program every few weeks "shocks" your muscles and advances your progress. It also keeps your exercise regimen fresh and interesting.

Of the four stand-alone workouts, the basic workout is the only one that uses the traditional movement patterns described in Chapter Eleven. If you're new to weight training, I recommend you start with the basic workout. The other three stand-alone workouts intensify the exercises by using non-traditional movement patterns.

The combo workouts offer more variety and higher intensity levels. Using two of the three different non-traditional movement patterns to do each exercise is particularly challenging because they intensify one another.

STAND-ALONE WORKOUTS

Option 1: Basic Workout

In the basic workout, you perform the traditional movement pattern for each positive and negative rep. Starting with the basic workout will help you become accustomed to using proper form. But getting back to basics periodically is a good idea for everyone. It allows you to monitor your progress and make sure you haven't adopted any bad habits (i.e., improper form).

Option 2: High Velocity Workout

In the high velocity workout, you perform each positive rep with an "explosive" movement. That is, do the positive rep fast, but make sure you stop before locking out, as always. Include a momentary pause between the end of the negative rep and the beginning of the next fast positive rep. The pause prevents momentum from doing much of the work. Remember, only your positive reps are fast. Negative reps are always slow (five to six seconds to complete).

You may recall in the discussion about proper form that I stressed the importance of doing both the positive and negative rep slowly and smoothly. For the high velocity workout, it's okay to do a fast positive rep, as long as you keep your body in the proper position and don't lock out. You have to concentrate to avoid locking out when you're doing high velocity positive reps, especially when using lighter weights.

You can intensify this workout by doing very slow negative reps (ten to twelve seconds to complete).

Keep in mind, it may be difficult to move heavier weights quickly. Don't worry about the speed; just give it your best effort with proper form. Interestingly, research suggests that it is not so much the actual speed of the movement, but the intention to move explosively that increases the intensity. In other words, the benefits come from attempting the fast movements, even if the resulting movement is slow. ("Velocity Specificity of Resistance Training: Actual Movement Velocity Versus Intention to Move," Strength and Conditioning Journal, April 2006.)

Option 3: Subdivided Reps Workout

In a traditional positive rep, you go through the full ROM in a single, smooth movement. But in the subdivided reps workout, you divide the ROM into three equal parts, with momentary pauses between them. Thus the movement goes like this: lift-pause-lift-pause-lift-finish (before lockout). Then do a normal negative rep. The pause should last about a second. Try to cover an equal distance in each part as you go through the full ROM.

Subdividing reps and pausing increases the amount of time the muscles are under tension.

You can intensify the subdivided reps workout by doing subdivided reps in both directions (positive and negative).

It may be difficult or awkward to subdivide wrist curls, reverse wrist curls and calf raises into three parts because of their relatively short ROMs. For these exercises, I suggest pausing only once about half-way through each positive and negative rep.

Option 4: Stop and Hold Workout

In the stop and hold workout, you pause for three seconds after each positive rep, then do the negative rep. The pause increases the amount of time the muscles are under tension.

You can intensify this workout by doing very slow negative reps (ten to twelve seconds to complete).

NON-TRADITIONAL COMBOS

As I mentioned, the non-traditional movement patterns in the high velocity, subdivided reps, and stop and hold workouts shock the muscles and advance your progress. By combining any two of these three workouts, you further challenge your muscles and increase the intensity. Following is a description of each possible combination:

Option 1: High Velocity/Stop and Hold: Perform high velocity positive reps, stop and hold for three seconds, then do a normal negative rep.

Option 2: High Velocity/Subdivided Reps: Perform high velocity positive reps, then subdivide the negative reps.

Option 3: Stop and Hold/Subdivided Reps: Do traditional positive reps, stop and hold for three seconds, then do subdivided negative reps.

CARDIO/WEIGHT-TRAINING COMBOS

The following combo workouts combine cardiovascular endurance training and muscle strength and endurance training, increasing the intensity and effectiveness of both. This type of workout is also efficient because it allows you to integrate your cardio training and weight training into one workout. If you want a new challenge or you're short on time, the cardio/weight-training combo is for you.

In these workouts, you do one of the four stand-alone workouts described earlier, but you alternate the weight-training exercises with aerobic activity. Thus your options are as follows:

Option 1: Basic Workout/Aerobic Exercise

Option 2: High Velocity/Aerobic Exercise

Option 3: Subdivided Reps/Aerobic Exercise

Option 4: Stop and Hold/Aerobic Exercise

These workouts require some pre-planning because smooth transitions and continuous activity are important. Before you start, divide the twelve weight-training exercises into four groups of three exercises each. You also need to decide on your aerobic activity. You can use your favorite piece of aerobic equipment throughout the workout, or use two or three pieces of aerobic equipment. The workout will take between thirty and forty-five minutes, depending on the amount of time you spend on aerobic activity and the number of reps you're doing for each exercise. The workout is structured as follows:

(1) Five-minute aerobic warm-up

(2) First group of three weight-training exercises

(3) Two to four minutes of aerobic exercise

(4) Second group of three weight-training exercises

(5) Two to four minutes of aerobic exercise

(6) Third group of three weight-training exercises

(7) Two to four minutes of aerobic exercise

(8) Fourth group of three weight-training exercises

(9) Two minutes of aerobic exercise

(10) Three-minute aerobic cool-down

(11) Static stretching

Following is a sample cardio/weight-training combo workout:

(1) Warm up on a treadmill (five minutes)

(2) Leg press, calf raises, bench press

(3) Aerobic exercise on a recumbent bicycle (three or four minutes)

(4) Pec dec, crunches, four-part seated row

(5) Aerobic exercise on an elliptical (one or two minutes; the elliptical is more intense)

(6) Reverse crunches, shoulder press, triceps press-downs OR triceps extensions

(7) Aerobic exercise on an upright bicycle (three or four minutes)

(8) Biceps curls, wrist curls, reverse wrist curls

(9) Aerobic exercise on a treadmill (two minutes)

(10) Cool down on the treadmill (alternately reduce the speed and elevation for three minutes)

(11) Static stretching

* Note: If you add inner/outer-thigh pulls, one of your exercise groups will have four exercises instead of three.

As noted earlier, adding aerobic exercise to your muscle strength and endurance workouts increases the intensity of both. You may have to reduce the number of reps you do and the amount of weight you use in the stand-alone workouts, at least initially. Keep in mind, since each aerobic exercise portion lasts only two to four minutes, you may not be able to use the IAT method described in the previous section. (To create your customized workout regimen, use the instructions and worksheets provided in Appendix Two.)

Section V

Static Stretching for Flexibility

Chapter Thirteen

Flexibility Is Freedom

Even if you don't have a physically demanding job, you probably spend much of your day moving. Throughout our daily lives we walk, reach and bend. Our muscles are often called on to act quickly.

The quality of your movements is determined by your degree of flexibility. The more flexible you are, the more efficient your movements. Engaging in static stretching will enhance your flexibility and help you avoid injury from physical activity as well as everyday movements.

In this chapter I'll tell you why flexibility is beneficial, what factors impede flexibility, and when you should stretch. In the following chapter I'll give you detailed instructions for safely and effectively stretching all the muscles you worked.

The Benefits of Static Stretching for Flexibility

Everyday movements, many of which are repetitive, can be uncomfortable or even painful if you lack flexibility. But if you're flexible, you can move freely and smoothly through full ranges of motion.

Static stretching increases your ROM around joints. It's the safest way to increase your flexibility because you control each stretch.

Increasing your ROM will improve your performance in sports and other recreational activities. Flexibility enhances your ability to use proper form when weight training. In addition, it reduces your risk of injury when you engage in physical activity.

Static stretching is often used to increase ROM after an injury or surgery—a testament to its benefits.

The next time you have to quickly reach over to catch that priceless vase that was accidentally knocked off the shelf, you'll be thankful you incorporated stretching into your exercise regimen.

Impediments to Flexibility

(1) Failure to Stretch

The main reason people lack flexibility is they don't stretch after engaging in strenuous physical activity, including weight training. Static stretching after physical activity elongates muscles, enhancing flexibility.

(2) Sedentary Lifestyle

If you never engage in any physical activity, your muscles will start to deteriorate due to lack of use. Muscles thrive on hard work. Without it, they gradually lose their elasticity and become shorter. This leads to soreness when you engage in routine tasks, such as getting out of bed in the morning or getting out of the car after a long drive.

(3) Excess Fat Accumulation

Excess fat obstructs movement. It acts as a physical barrier, limiting how close one bone can get to another bone when muscles contract. Simple tasks such as bending over to pick something up or raising a foot to put on a sock become more difficult. The movements are restricted. But stretching alone will not address this problem. As I've stressed before, engaging in all four components of The Awesome Foursome is the most effective and safest way to lose excess fat.

(4) Genetics

Of the four impediments to flexibility, genetics is the only one you can't control. Your genetic makeup determines your body type, the length of your muscles and tendons, and the number of different muscle fibers. While you can't change your genetic make-up, you can take action that will have an impact on your genetic predispositions.

Always Stretch *After* Your Workout

Stretching Is Not a Warm-up

You've probably seen people stretch before engaging in a physical activity, such as running or tennis. When a muscle has rested for a period of time, it's "cold." Stretching a cold muscle is unproductive and even dangerous for the following reasons:

- Cold muscles cannot achieve their full ranges of motion.
- Stretching a cold muscle can lead to injury.

Think of it this way: muscles and tendons are elastic like rubber bands. If you put a rubber band in the freezer for a period of time, and then try to stretch it, it will break. Similarly, if you stretch a cold muscle, it can be difficult and painful. You may even strain or tear it.

Stretching before engaging in physical activity increases your risk of injury during the activity. If you succeed in partially elongating a muscle by stretching it and then make an explosive movement, the muscle is forcibly pulled beyond its limit.

A number of recent research studies have found that warming up by statically stretching before weight training, playing a sport, or engaging in any strenuous physical activity adversely affects performance, strength and power, which can increase the risk of injury.

As you know from reading the section on muscle strength and endurance training, aerobic exercise is a fast and effective way to warm up your muscles before lifting weights or engaging in any other strenuous physical activity. Aerobic exercise increases your heart rate, causing it to pump more blood around your body. Blood brings warmth to muscles. Warm muscles are less likely to be torn or strained because they are more supple.

Stretching Is a Cool-down

The time to stretch is after you engage in physical activity, such as your cardio or weight-training workout, when muscles are warm and supple. Stretching after your workout routine has the following benefits:

- Increases the range of motion around joints.
- Serves as a cool-down.

- Enhances your performance in sports and other recreational activities.
- Prevents injuries.
- May decrease muscle recovery time.

Chapter Fourteen

Facilitating Flexibility

In this chapter you'll find instructions for safely and effectively stretching after your workouts. (After you thoroughly familiarize yourself with these instructions, you can consult the quick reference charts in Appendix Three for a handy reminder.) The instructions are accompanied by illustrations. Before going over the stretches, let's talk about the proper form for stretching and the stretching routine.

Proper Form Is Critical

Using proper form when you're stretching is essential for achieving positive results and avoiding injury. When stretching, adhere to the following guidelines:

- **Do not bounce.** Bouncing up and down or side to side when stretching is unproductive and can cause muscle strains and tears. I use the term "static stretching" to indicate that you remain still during the stretch.

- **Stretch slowly.** Get into each stretch position slowly, and come out of it slowly.
- **Hold the stretch.** Instead of bouncing, you should hold the stretch for fifteen or twenty seconds.
- **Relax your muscles**. When you stop and hold a stretch, relax the muscle you're stretching. Don't fight against the stretch. Also, relax muscles that are not being stretched.

The Stretching Routine

I've provided stretches for the muscles that you worked based on the previous section. Do only one stretch, one time, for each muscle (holding each stretch for fifteen to twenty seconds). In some cases, you'll find more than one stretch for a muscle. Do the one that's most comfortable for you, or alternate from workout to workout. I also provide stretches that benefit more than one muscle.

The order in which you do the stretches is up to you. Find a flow that you're comfortable with. However, you may find it easier to start your stretching routine standing up. After you do all of the standing stretches, sit on the mat for the sitting stretches, and finally lie down for the rest of the stretches. If you prefer, you can reverse the order (lie down on the mat, sit, stand).

Stretching is not just for your workouts. You should go through your entire stretching routine after engaging in any strenuous physical activity, from shoveling snow to painting the house. As long as you've increased your heart rate and your muscles are warmed up, it's safe and beneficial to stretch.

On days when you do only a cardio workout, you should at least stretch your lower back and legs (quads, hams and calves).

If you see or feel the muscle being stretched quiver or "flutter" at any time during the stretch, back off slowly. But as I mentioned in the previous section, pain is a warning sign. If you feel pain while stretching, STOP immediately.

THE STRETCHES

Lower Back

Option One

(1) Lie on your back with your knees bent and your feet flat on a mat.

(2) Bring one knee toward your chest.

(3) Clasp your hands (interlock your fingers with your palms facing each other) around the hamstrings (back of the upper leg) in the bend behind the kneecap, or clasp your hands, with an interlocking grip, around your lower leg just below the kneecap.

(4) Pull your knee toward your chest until you feel a stretch in your lower back. Stop and hold.

(5) Repeat with your other leg.

(See Figure 21)

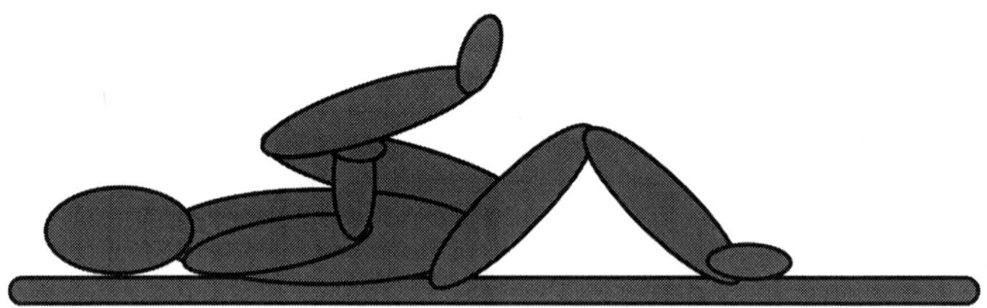

Figure 21: Lower Back Stretch (Option One)

Lower Back

Option Two

(1) Lie on your back with your knees bent and your feet flat on the mat.
(2) Bring both bent knees toward your chest.
(3) Put one hand around each leg just below the kneecap or put both arms around both legs (hug them) just below the kneecaps.
(4) Pull both knees toward your chest until you feel the stretch in your lower back. Stop and hold.

(See Figure 22)

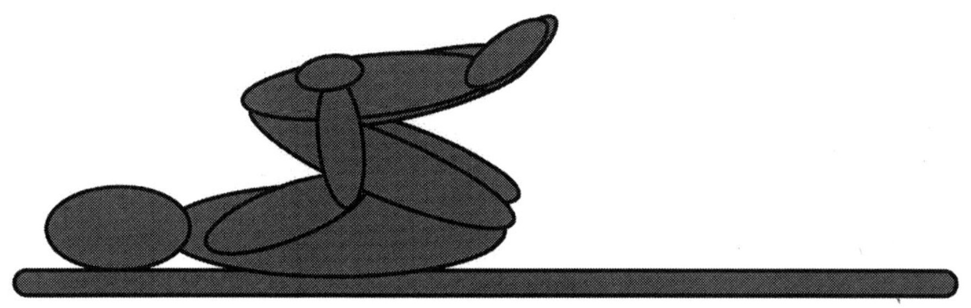

Figure 22: Lower Back Stretch (Option Two)

Quads (front of thigh)

Option One

(1) Lie on your left side.

(2) Extend your left arm out (palm on mat) to form a 90 degree angle with your trunk. The extended arm helps maintain balance.

(3) Bend your right leg.

(4) Grasp your right ankle with your right hand.

(5) Bring your right heel as close to your buttocks as possible while keeping your legs parallel. Stop and hold.

(6) Repeat on your right side with your right arm extended out.

(See Figure 23)

* Note: If you can't bend your leg up far enough to grab your ankle, try Option Two.

* Note: It's essential that you keep your legs parallel. Never move or pull the leg being stretched away from the straight leg. This can strain the groin muscles and put stress on the knee joint.

* Note: The shoulder of the extended arm can be used as a head-rest. If this is uncomfortable, fold a towel into a small pillow or roll it into a bolster to fill in the curve in your neck.

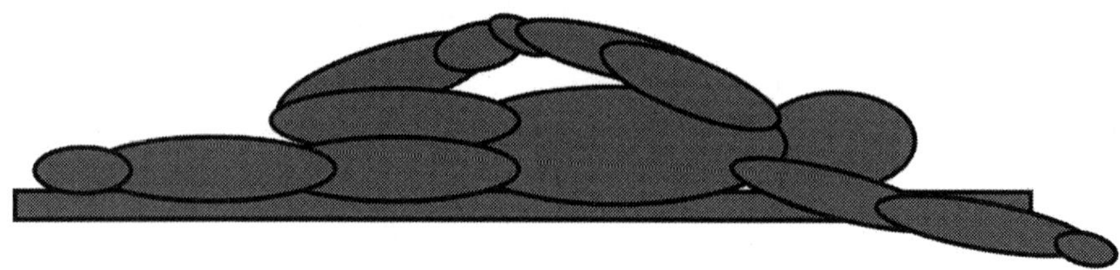

Figure 23: Quad Stretch (Option One)

Quads (front of thigh)

Option Two

(1) Place an object on the floor behind you to serve as a foot rest (e.g., a step stool) or use either the bottom or second step of a staircase.

(2) Stand up straight but don't lock out your knees.

(3) If necessary, brace (balance) yourself by placing your right hand on the back of a chair, for example. Use the railing if your foot is on a step.

(4) Bend your right knee and place your toes on the foot rest. Keep your legs parallel. If they're not, reposition the object or yourself until your legs are parallel.

(5) Make sure the object is high enough for you to feel a stretch in the quads (front of thigh). Stop and hold.

(6) Repeat with your left leg, bracing yourself with your left hand, if necessary.

(See Figure 24)

* Note: As your flexibility improves, you will be able to put your foot on higher objects. Eventually, you'll be able to raise it high enough to grab your ankle with your hand. At that point, you can do Option One or Option Three.

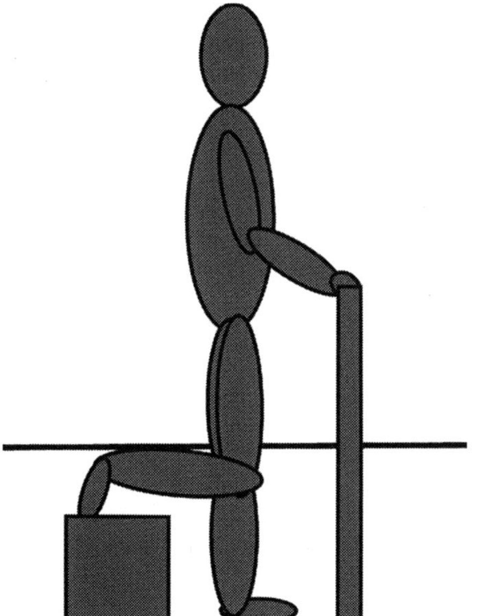

Figure 24: Quad Stretch (Option Two)

Quads (front of thigh)

Option Three

(1) Stand up straight but don't lock out your knees.

(2) If necessary, brace (balance) yourself by placing your left hand on the back of a chair, for example.

(3) Bend your right leg.

(4) Grasp your right ankle with your right hand.

(5) Bring your heel as close to your buttocks as possible. Keep your legs parallel. Stop and hold.

(6) Repeat with the left leg bracing yourself with your right hand.

(See Figure 25)

* Note: Make sure that your legs are parallel. Never move or pull the leg being stretched away from the leg you're standing on. This can strain the groin muscles and put stress on the knee joint.

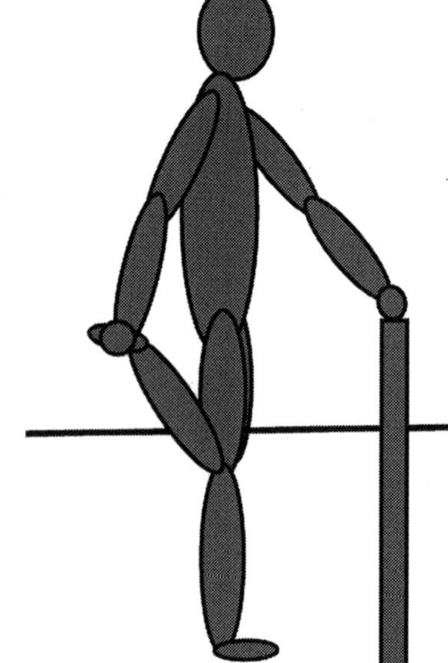

Figure 25: Quad Stretch (Option Three)

Hams (back of thigh)

Option One

(1) Sit on a mat with your legs extended straight out and together and your toes pointed toward the ceiling. Your feet and ankles form 90 degree angles.

(2) Bend from the waist and grasp any part of your legs, from the ankles on up, that you can reach.

(3) Aim your chin toward your knees.

(4) Stop and hold the position at which you feel a stretch in your hams (back of thighs).

(See Figure 26)

* Note: Always bend and reach out slowly to grasp your legs and anchor yourself.

* Note: To increase the stretch, bend your arms and lower your elbows. This may enable you to get your chest a bit closer to your knees. Keeping your arms straight restricts movement.

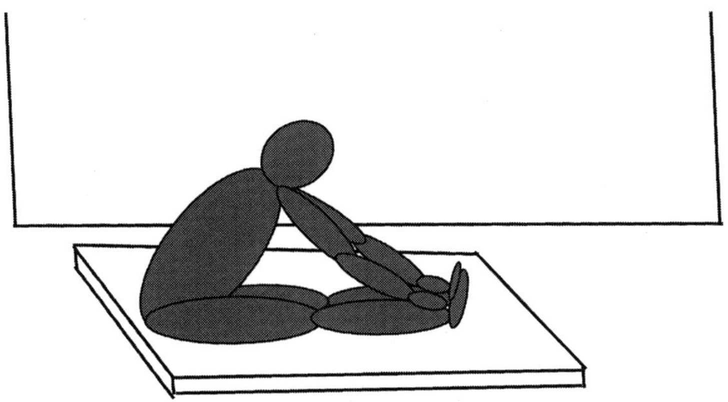

Figure 26: Hams Stretch (Option One)

Hams (back of thigh)

Option Two

(1) Place an object on the floor in front of you to serve as a foot rest (e.g., a step stool) or use either the bottom or second step of a staircase.

(2) If necessary, brace (balance) yourself by placing your left hand on the back of a chair, for example. You can use the railing if you're using a step.

(3) Keeping your left leg straight, lift it and place your heel on the foot rest.

(4) Make sure the object you use is high enough for you to feel a stretch in your hams. Stop and hold.

(5) Repeat with the right leg, bracing yourself with your right hand.

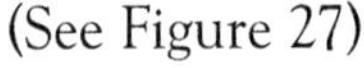

(See Figure 27)

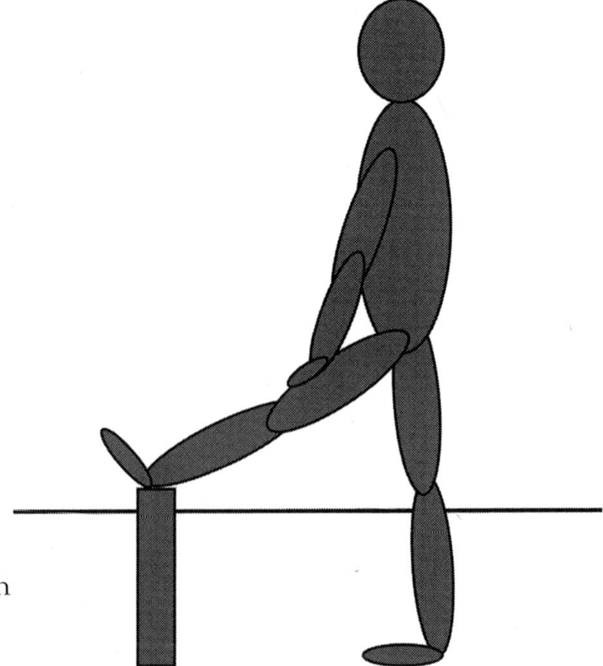

Figure 27: Hams Stretch (Option Two)

Option Two–Modifications

If you've completed steps (1) through (3) and you don't feel a stretch, but you cannot get your leg up higher, try the following:

(4) Place and rest your left hand on your left thigh, bracing yourself with your right hand, if necessary.

(5) Keeping your torso straight, lean in (bending from the waist). Slide your left hand down your thigh as you lean in. When you feel a stretch in your hams, stop and hold.

(6) Repeat with the right leg, bracing yourself with your left hand, if necessary.

If you don't have to brace yourself by holding on to anything, do the following:

(4) Place both hands on your left thigh, one on top of the other.

(5) Slowly lean in (bending from your waist) as you slide your hands down your leg. As soon as you feel a stretch in your hams, stop and hold.

(6) Repeat with right leg.

Calves

Option One

(1) Stand about six inches away from a wall with your feet about shoulder width apart.

(2) Place your hands on the wall at about eye level.

(3) Move one foot back as far as you can and still keep the heel of that foot firmly planted on the floor.

(4) The other leg will be bent at about 90 degrees at the knee.

(5) If you feel a stretch in the calf (the back of the lower leg) that is behind you, hold that position. If not, lean in toward the wall slowly until you do feel a stretch.

(6) Stop and hold.

(7) Repeat with the other leg.

(See Figure 28, image on left)

* Note: If the heel of the foot that's behind you comes up and off the floor, the stretch is compromised. If you have to, move that leg a bit closer to the wall.

Option Two

(1) Stand about a foot away from a wall with your feet about shoulder width apart.

(2) Place your hands on the wall at about eye level.

(3) Keep one leg straight but not locked out.

(4) Place the heel of the other foot on the floor as close to the wall as possible by getting the ball of that foot up on the wall.

(5) If you feel a stretch in your calf, hold that position. If you don't,

lean in slowly toward the wall until you do.

(6) Stop and hold.
(7) Repeat with the other leg.

(See Figure 28, image on right)

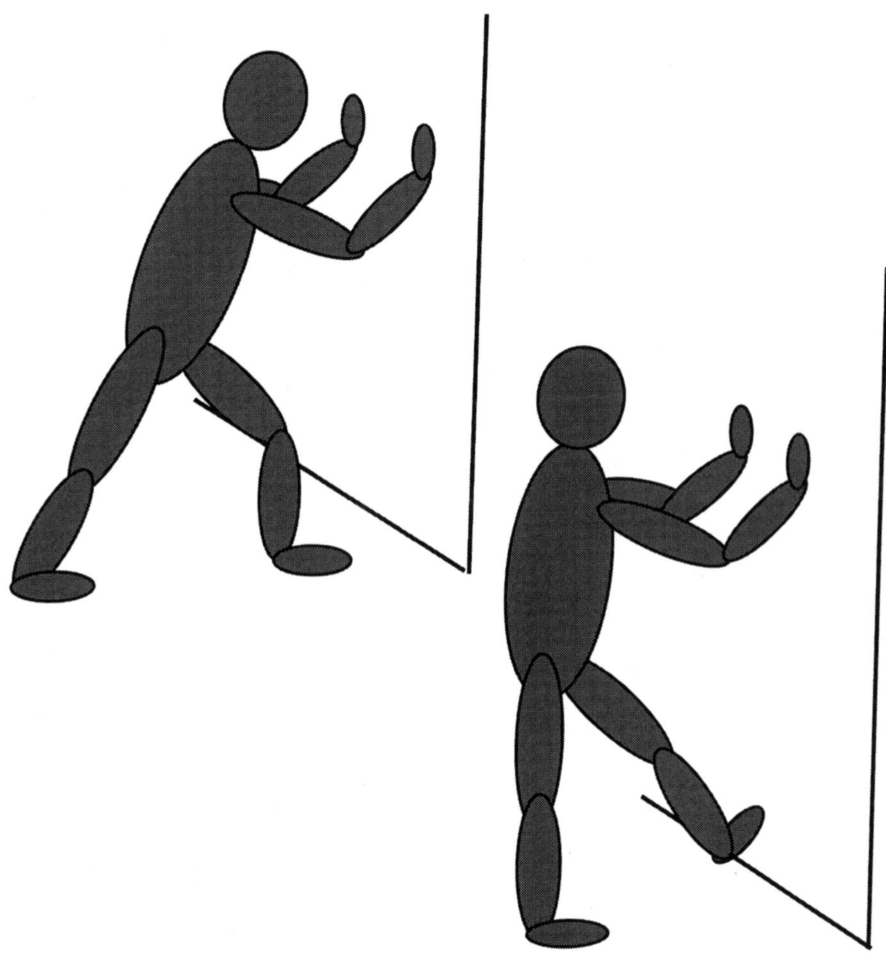

Figure 28: Calf Stretch (Options One and Two)

Inner Thighs

* Note: Do this stretch only if you do inner/outer thigh pulls.

(1) Sit with your back against a wall.

(2) Bend both legs at the knees.

(3) Bring the soles of your feet as close together as possible.

(4) Grasp your ankles and gently pull your feet as close to your body as possible. Your legs will form a diamond shape. Rest your hands on your lap.

(5) If you feel a stretch in your inner thighs (groin). Stop and hold.

(See Figure 29)

<u>Modification</u>

If you don't feel the stretch, do the following:

(1) Place your hands on your knees.

(2) Gently and slowly try to move your knees down slightly.

(3) As soon as you feel a stretch, stop and hold.

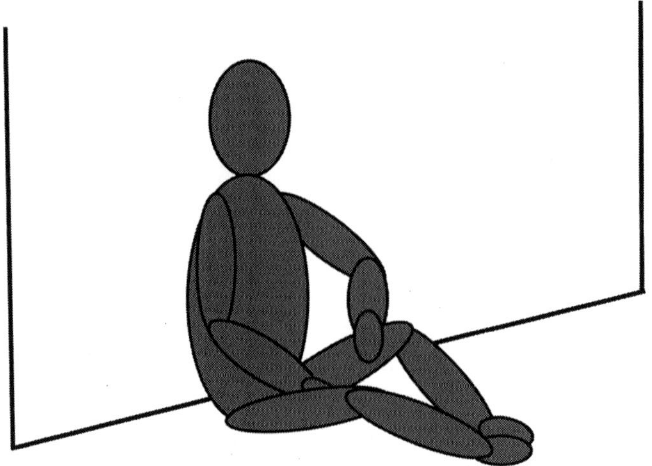

Figure 29: Inner Thighs Stretch

Outer Thighs, Sides and Lower Back

* Note: Do this stretch only if you do inner/outer thigh pulls. However, this stretch is also good for the sides and lower back.

(1) Sit on a mat with your left leg extended.

(2) Bend your right leg and place your right foot on the floor at the outside of your left knee so that the foot touches the knee.

(3) Put your right hand on the floor about a foot behind you in line with your right hip.

(4) Sit with your upper body making as close to a 90 degree angle with your hips as possible.

(5) Put your left elbow against the outside of your right leg at the bend of your knee.

(6) Slowly rotate your upper body and your head to the right.

(7) Slowly and gently push your right leg to the left with your left elbow.

(8) When you feel a stretch in the muscles on the outside of your right hip, lower back and sides, stop and hold.

(9) Repeat on the other side (extend the right leg and bend the left).

(See Figure 30)

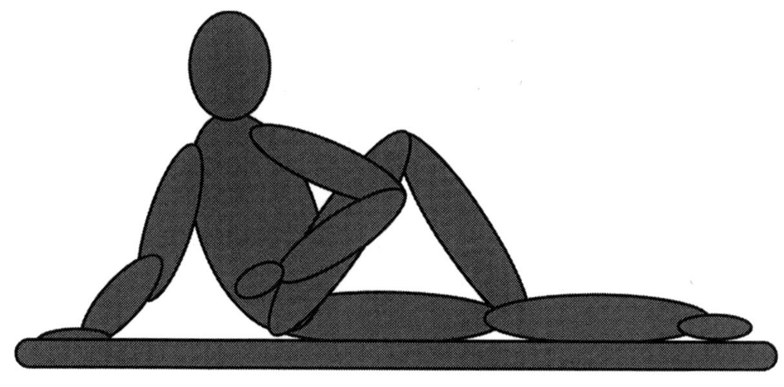

Figure 30: Outer Thighs, Sides and Lower Back

Shoulders, Upper Back and Triceps

(1) Stand up straight. Extend one arm across your body just under your chin.

(2) Place the palm of your other hand on the elbow of the extended arm.

(3) If you feel a stretch in the back of your shoulder, upper back and triceps, stop and hold.

(4) If you don't feel a stretch, gently push your elbow in toward your chest until you do.

(5) Repeat with your other arm.

(See Figure 31, image on left)

* Note: You have the option of bending the extended arm at about a 90 degree angle at the elbow. Gently push your elbow in toward your chest so that your hand goes over your shoulder and behind you.

Shoulders and Chest

(1) Stand straight with your feet about shoulder width apart.

(2) Extend your arms straight down behind you and clasp your hands (interlock your fingers so that your palms face each other).

(3) If you feel a stretch in the front of your shoulders and across your chest, hold that position. If you don't, slowly and gently raise your extended arms up until you do feel a stretch. Keep your shoulders straight and don't shrug them.

(See Figure 31, image on right)

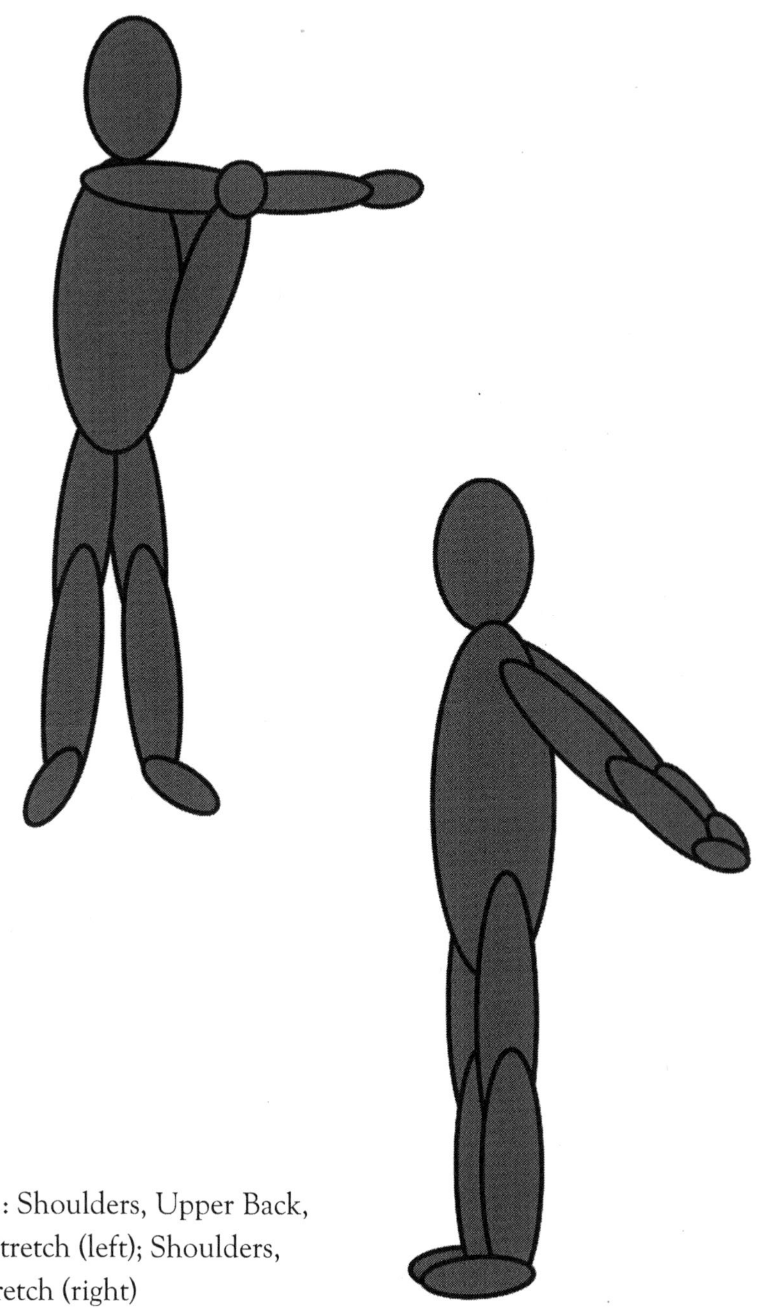

Figure 31: Shoulders, Upper Back, Triceps Stretch (left); Shoulders, Chest Stretch (right)

Forearms

(1) Stand straight with your legs about shoulder width apart.

(2) Extend your arms straight out in front of you at or a bit below shoulder level.

(3) Rotate both hands so that your palms are facing up and your thumbs are pointing out. Stop and hold.

(4) Rotate both hands so that the backs of your hands face each other and your thumbs point down. Stop and hold.

(5) Bend your right wrist so that your fingers point down and the palm faces you.

(6) Place your left hand across the back of your right hand.

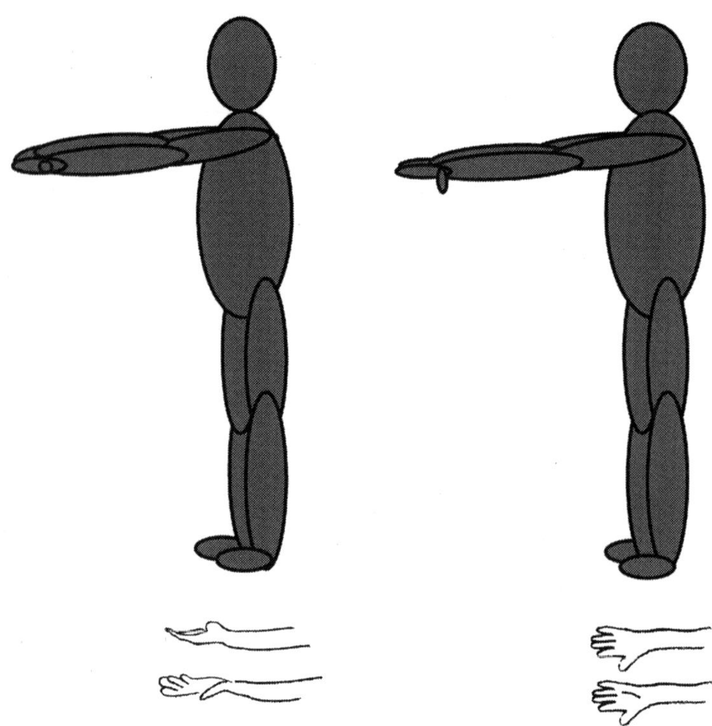

Figure 32: Forearms Stretch

(7) Gently pull your right hand toward you until you feel a stretch in the muscles along the top of your forearm. Stop and hold.

(8) Bend your right wrist so that your fingers point down and your palm faces away from you.

(9) Place your left hand across the four fingers of your right hand.

(10) Gently pull your right hand toward you until you feel a stretch in the muscles along the bottom of your forearm. Stop and hold.

(11) Repeat steps 5 through 9 with your left hand.

(See Figure 32)

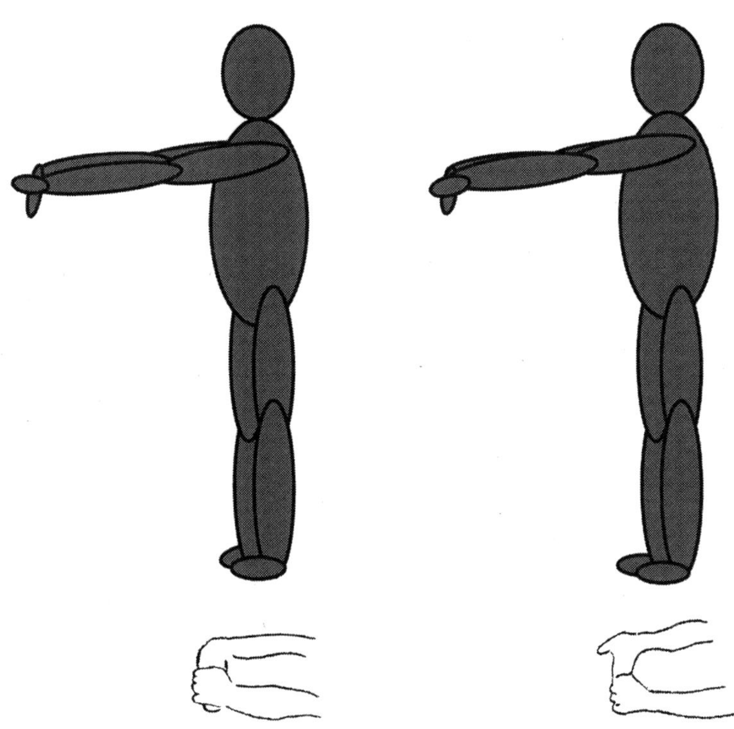

Upper Back and Sides

(1) Stand straight with your feet about shoulder width apart.

(2) Raise your arms above your head.

(3) Grasp your right wrist with your left hand.

(4) Bend your elbows slightly.

(5) Bend over from your waist to the left while slowly and gently pulling your right arm to the left. Stop and hold.

(6) Repeat with your right hand gently pulling your left arm to the right.

(See Figure 33, image on left)

* Note: If you're uncomfortable bending with your arms over your head, you can do the following stretch for your sides. Keep in mind this position doesn't stretch your upper back.

Sides

(1) Stand with your feet about shoulder width apart.

(2) Keep your arms at your sides.

(3) Bend (lean) from your waist to the right. Your right hand will slide down your side and your left hand will slide up. Relax your arms. Keep your shoulders straight. Don't slouch and don't shrug your shoulders.

(4) Repeat on the other side.

(See Figure 33, image on right)

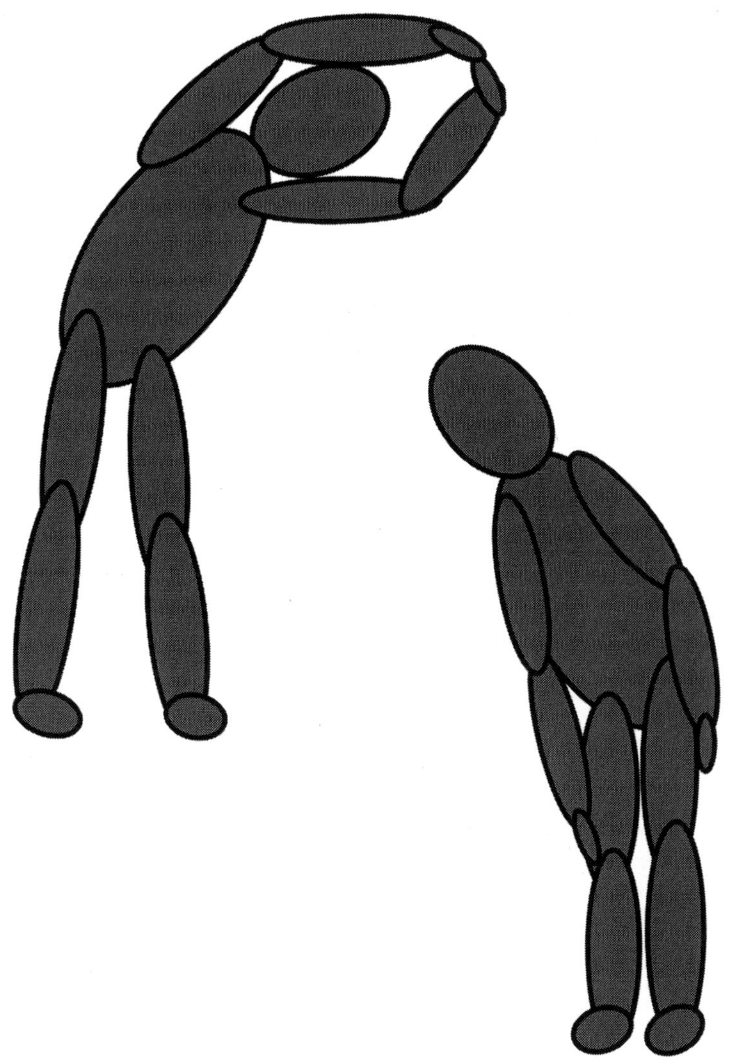

Figure 33: Upper Back and Sides Stretch (left),
Sides Stretch (right)

Summary

We can't stop the aging process. But proper nutrition and regular exercise can prolong your life and improve the quality of your life. The Awesome Foursome gives you the tools to transform your body and enjoy an active lifestyle. Following is a recap of the key points discussed in this book:

A sensible eating lifestyle focuses on health, not weight.

- Increase your awareness of what you eat and the potential effects on your health; you're likely to make better choices.
- You can't attain your long-term goal of optimal health and total fitness through dieting, and the potential risks associated with dieting exceed their supposed benefits.
- Eat more complex carbohydrates (whole grains) because they supply fuel for your body and fill you up, reducing your urge to binge on junk food.

- Reduce your consumption of sugar and salt, which have negative health effects.
- Eat more fruits and vegetables, which contain an assortment of important vitamins, minerals and antioxidants.
- A sensible eating lifestyle is not about deprivation. It's about making good choices most of the time, while still allowing yourself the occasional indulgence.

Cardiovascular (C/V) endurance training (regular aerobic exercise) increases the efficiency of your cardiovascular system, enabling you to engage in physical activity for longer periods of time without fatiguing. It also wards off certain medical conditions, and enhances your brain functioning.

- Engage in aerobic exercise for thirty minutes (including your warm-up and cool-down) three times a week.
- Get your heart rate into your target zone gradually by engaging in a five- to ten-minute warm-up.
- Keep your heart rate in its target zone for twenty minutes.
- Decrease your heart rate gradually by engaging in a five-minute cool-down. Never abruptly stop your aerobic activity.

Muscle strength and endurance training will not only improve your performance in sports and other physical activities, but it will also make your daily activities easier and reduce your risk of injury.

- Muscles that are strong and toned burn more calories even when at rest than do muscles that are not developed.
- One-set workouts are more efficient than multiple set workouts

because they take less time. They're also safer and reduce the risk of injury.

- Your muscles require a "rest period" of at least twenty-four hours between workouts.
- To work out safely and achieve results, you must adhere to proper form.
- Engage in aerobic exercise for five to ten minutes before weight training to warm up your muscles.
- Follow your workout with a cool-down period that consists of static stretching. Never statically stretch before engaging in any physical activity because stretching a "cold" muscle increases the risk of injury.
- Do your weight-training workout three times a week.

Engaging in static stretching will enhance your flexibility and help you avoid injury from physical activity as well as everyday movements.

- Stretching is not a warm-up. Stretching a cold muscle is unproductive and dangerous.
- Stretch after you engage in physical activity, such as your cardiovascular or weight-training workout, when muscles are warm and supple.
- Do not bounce when stretching. Bouncing up and down or side to side when stretching is unproductive and can cause muscle strains and tears.

Important medical information:

- Consult your doctor before starting a new exercise regimen or changing your current one.
- Stop exercising if you feel pain and seek medical attention
- Stop exercising if you feel nauseous, light-headed or dizzy, or you have chest pain or tightness in your chest. Seek medical attention.

The Awesome Foursome is not a short-term program for losing weight or sculpting your body. It's a lifestyle. If you make a commitment to incorporate sensible eating, aerobic exercise, weight-training and static stretching into your lifestyle—for the rest of your life—you will attain more than a better physique. You will improve your overall health and enjoy a better quality of life.

Author's Note

Please visit www.awesomefoursomebook.com for more information and to download useful reference guides and worksheets.

About the Author

Dr. Irwin Schwartz, Ed.D., CSCS, is a health and fitness professional with more than thirty-five years of experience in the field. He created the curriculum for the Wellness and Physical Fitness course at Pace University (Pleasantville, NY) in 2000, and has been teaching the course since then.

In 1999, Dr. Schwartz entered an Athletic Training Internship Program and completed more than 1,500 clinical hours in sports medicine. He worked with college athletes and was involved in the assessment, treatment, rehabilitation and prevention of their sports injuries. In 2000, he earned his Certification as a Strength and Conditioning Specialist (CSCS) from the National Strength and Conditioning Association (NSCA). In 2008, he became a professional member of the American College of Sports Medicine (ACSM).

While working as a personal trainer and fitness consultant from 1982 to 2000, Dr. Schwartz wrote and produced two instructional videos and a manual on the safe and proper use of home weight-training equipment.

From 1982 to 1991, Dr. Schwartz co-owned and operated Exercise Guidance Associates, Inc. in Chappaqua, NY, where he and his partner sold exercise equipment, designed total fitness programs for their clients, and supervised their workouts.

Before joining the faculty at Pace, Dr. Schwartz had worked at Arturo Toscanini Community Junior High School 145 in the Bronx since 1968. He served as an assistant principal, health and physical education instructor, team leader, health coordinator and coach.

Dr. Schwartz attained a Doctor of Education degree in 1976 from Fordham University. He earned a Master of Science in Health from Herbert H. Lehman College in 1970. In 1968, he received a Bachelor of Arts in Physical Education from Hunter College, where he minored in physiology and anatomy.

At age sixty-five, Dr. Schwartz continues to play baseball in a thirty-five and up league. The 2009 baseball season marked his fifty-first consecutive season playing organized baseball or fast pitch softball. He coaches youth baseball and basketball.

Dr. Schwartz has expertise in the physiology of muscular activity, the physiology of exercise, physiology and anatomy, kinesiology, the efficiency of human movement, and sports medicine. He has advised or personally trained people ranging in age from fourteen to eighty-nine, including those with various medical and physical problems and unique limitations and constraints. He gives presentations on health and fitness to community groups.

Appendix One

Food Diary

Day One

Breakfast: ____________________________

Snack: ____________________________

Lunch: ____________________________

Snack: ____________________________

Dinner: ____________________________

Snack: ____________________________

2 Day Two

Breakfast: ______________________________

Snack: ______________________________

Lunch: ______________________________

Snack: ______________________________

Dinner: ______________________________

Snack: ______________________________

3 Day Three

Breakfast: ______________________________

Snack: ______________________________

Lunch: ______________________________

Snack: ______________________________

Dinner: ______________________________

Snack: ______________________________

Appendix Two

Create Your Workout Regimen In Five Easy Steps

Step One: Select an Aerobic Activity

Options

- Walking, jogging or running on a treadmill, on an inside track, on an outside track, in a recreational area or park, around your block or neighborhood.
- Step-ups (stepping up and down on the bottom step of a stairway inside or outside your home, or on equipment designed for step-ups).
- Swimming laps in an indoor or outdoor pool.
- Riding your bicycle around the block, on a bike trail, or on a scenic tour.

- Riding a stationary bicycle in your home or at the gym.
- Roller blading or roller skating.
- Cross country skiing.
- Any other continuous, non-competitive physical activity that elevates your heart rate.

Step Two: Select a Weight Training Workout Program

Options

Stand-alone Workouts

- Basic
- High Velocity
- Subdivided Reps
- Stop and Hold

Non-Traditional Combos

- High Velocity/Stop and Hold
- High Velocity/Subdivided Reps
- Stop and Hold/Subdivided Rep

Cardio/Weight-Training Combos

- Basic Workout/Aerobic Exercise
- High Velocity/Aerobic Exercise
- Subdivided Reps/Aerobic Exercise
- Stop and Hold/Aerobic Exercise

Step Three: Select a Weight Training Workout Routine

Options

Workout Routine One

(1) Leg Press

(2) Bench Press

(3) Calf Raises

(4) Pec Dec

(5) Crunches

(6) Four-part Seated Row

(7) Reverse Crunches

(8) Shoulder Press

(9) Triceps Press-downs OR Triceps Extensions

(10) Biceps Curls

(11) Wrist Curls

(12) Reverse Wrist Curls

Workout Routine Two

(1) Leg Extensions

(2) Bench Press

(3) Leg Curls

(4) Pec Dec

(5) Calf Raises

(6) Four-part Seated Row

(7) Combo Crunches

(8) Shoulder Press

(9) Triceps Press-downs OR Triceps Extensions

(10) Biceps Curls

(11) Wrist Curls

(12) Reverse Wrist Curls

Step Four: Determine Reps and Weights

Options

Strength Workout

Use heavier weights and do fewer reps.

Find a weight for each exercise that you can lift between four and eight times.

Local Muscular Endurance Workout

Use lighter weights and do more reps.

Find a weight for each exercise that you can lift between fourteen and eighteen times.

Step Five: Develop a Schedule

Options

(1) Thirty-minute cardio workout, followed by weight training workout, three times a week

Sample Schedule

Monday: Cardio workout, weight training workout
Tuesday: Rest
Wednesday: Cardio workout, weight training workout
Thursday: Rest
Friday: Cardio workout, weight training workout
Saturday: Rest
Sunday: Rest

(2) Alternate cardio workouts and weight training workouts during the week

Sample Schedule

Monday: Cardio workout
Tuesday: Weight training workout
Wednesday: Cardio workout
Thursday: Weight training workout
Friday: Cardio workout
Saturday: Weight training workout
Sunday: Rest

(3) Cardio/weight training combo workout three times a week

Sample Schedule

Monday: Rest
Tuesday: Combo workout
Wednesday: Rest
Thursday: Combo workout
Friday: Rest
Saturday: Rest
Sunday: Combo workout

(4) Stretched Out Workout Week

Sample Schedule

Monday: Cardio workout
Tuesday: Weight training workout
Wednesday: Rest
Thursday: Cardio workout
Friday: Weight training workout

Saturday: Rest
Sunday: Rest
Monday: Cardio workout
Tuesday: Weight training workout

* **Important Reminder:** Begin every workout with a five-minute warm-up, and end every workout with a cool-down that consists of static stretching. If you do a total body weight training workout, go through your entire stretching routine. If you do only a cardio workout, at least stretch your lower back and legs afterward.

* **Important Reminder:** Rotate among the different workouts programs and alternate between the two workout routines. Also alternate between local muscular endurance workouts and strength workouts, which will change the number of reps you do and the amount of weight you use. You can also rotate among different aerobic exercises.

On the following pages I've provided worksheets you can use to plan your workout schedule over the course of a month, and record the number of reps and amount of weight you will use for each exercise.

My Workout Regimen

Week One

Monday:

Aerobic Activity ________________________________

Weight Training Workout Program ______________________

Weight Training Workout Routine ______________________

Or Rest

Tuesday:

Aerobic Activity ________________________________

Weight Training Workout Program ______________________

Weight Training Workout Routine ______________________

Or Rest

Wednesday:

Aerobic Activity ________________________________

Weight Training Workout Program ______________________

Weight Training Workout Routine ______________________

Or Rest

Thursday:

Aerobic Activity ________________________________

Weight Training Workout Program ______________________

Weight Training Workout Routine ______________________

Or Rest

Friday:

Aerobic Activity ____________________

Weight Training Workout Program ____________________

Weight Training Workout Routine ____________________

Or Rest

Saturday:

Aerobic Activity ____________________

Weight Training Workout Program ____________________

Weight Training Workout Routine ____________________

Or Rest

Sunday:

Aerobic Activity ____________________

Weight Training Workout Program ____________________

Weight Training Workout Routine ____________________

Or Rest

Workout Routine One	Reps	Weight
Leg Press		
Bench Press		
Calf Raises		
Pec Dec		
Crunches *		
Four-part Seated Row		
Reverse Crunches		NA
Shoulder Press		
Triceps Press-downs		
OR Triceps Extensions		
Biceps Curls		
Wrist Curls		
Reverse Wrist Curls		

* Note the weight only if you do crunches on an ab crunch machine. If you do crunches on a mat, leave the weight line blank.

Workout Routine Two	Reps	Weight
Leg Extentions		
Bench Press		
Leg Curls		
Pec Dec		
Calf Raises		
Four-part Seated Row		
Combo Crunches		NA
Shoulder Press		
Triceps Press-downs		
OR Triceps Extensions		
Biceps Curls		
Wrist Curls		
Reverse Wrist Curls		

My Workout Regimen

Week Two

Monday:

Aerobic Activity ______________________________

Weight Training Workout Program______________________

Weight Training Workout Routine______________________

Or Rest

Tuesday:

Aerobic Activity ______________________________

Weight Training Workout Program______________________

Weight Training Workout Routine______________________

Or Rest

Wednesday:

Aerobic Activity ______________________________

Weight Training Workout Program______________________

Weight Training Workout Routine______________________

Or Rest

Thursday:

Aerobic Activity ______________________________

Weight Training Workout Program______________________

Weight Training Workout Routine______________________

Or Rest

Friday:

Aerobic Activity ______________________________

Weight Training Workout Program ______________________________

Weight Training Workout Routine ______________________________

Or Rest

Saturday:

Aerobic Activity ______________________________

Weight Training Workout Program ______________________________

Weight Training Workout Routine ______________________________

Or Rest

Sunday:

Aerobic Activity ______________________________

Weight Training Workout Program ______________________________

Weight Training Workout Routine ______________________________

Or Rest

Workout Routine One	Reps	Weight
Leg Press		
Bench Press		
Calf Raises		
Pec Dec		
Crunches *		
Four-part Seated Row		
Reverse Crunches		NA
Shoulder Press		
Triceps Press-downs		
OR Triceps Extensions		
Biceps Curls		
Wrist Curls		
Reverse Wrist Curls		

* Note the weight only if you do crunches on an ab crunch machine. If you do crunches on a mat, leave the weight line blank.

Workout Routine Two	Reps	Weight
Leg Extentions		
Bench Press		
Leg Curls		
Pec Dec		
Calf Raises		
Four-part Seated Row		
Combo Crunches		NA
Shoulder Press		
Triceps Press-downs		
OR Triceps Extensions		
Biceps Curls		
Wrist Curls		
Reverse Wrist Curls		

My Workout Regimen

Week Three

Monday:

Aerobic Activity ____________________

Weight Training Workout Program ____________________

Weight Training Workout Routine ____________________

Or Rest

Tuesday:

Aerobic Activity ____________________

Weight Training Workout Program ____________________

Weight Training Workout Routine ____________________

Or Rest

Wednesday:

Aerobic Activity ____________________

Weight Training Workout Program ____________________

Weight Training Workout Routine ____________________

Or Rest

Thursday:

Aerobic Activity ____________________

Weight Training Workout Program ____________________

Weight Training Workout Routine ____________________

Or Rest

Friday:

Aerobic Activity ______________________________

Weight Training Workout Program____________________

Weight Training Workout Routine____________________

Or Rest

Saturday:

Aerobic Activity ______________________________

Weight Training Workout Program____________________

Weight Training Workout Routine____________________

Or Rest

Sunday:

Aerobic Activity ______________________________

Weight Training Workout Program____________________

Weight Training Workout Routine____________________

Or Rest

Workout Routine One	Reps	Weight
Leg Press		
Bench Press		
Calf Raises		
Pec Dec		
Crunches *		
Four-part Seated Row		
Reverse Crunches		NA
Shoulder Press		
Triceps Press-downs		
OR Triceps Extensions		
Biceps Curls		
Wrist Curls		
Reverse Wrist Curls		

* Note the weight only if you do crunches on an ab crunch machine. If you do crunches on a mat, leave the weight line blank.

Workout Routine Two	Reps	Weight
Leg Extentions		
Bench Press		
Leg Curls		
Pec Dec		
Calf Raises		
Four-part Seated Row		
Combo Crunches		NA
Shoulder Press		
Triceps Press-downs		
OR Triceps Extensions		
Biceps Curls		
Wrist Curls		
Reverse Wrist Curls		

My Workout Regimen

Week Four

Monday:

Aerobic Activity ______________________________

Weight Training Workout Program____________________

Weight Training Workout Routine____________________

Or Rest

Tuesday:

Aerobic Activity ______________________________

Weight Training Workout Program____________________

Weight Training Workout Routine____________________

Or Rest

Wednesday:

Aerobic Activity ______________________________

Weight Training Workout Program____________________

Weight Training Workout Routine____________________

Or Rest

Thursday:

Aerobic Activity ______________________________

Weight Training Workout Program____________________

Weight Training Workout Routine____________________

Or Rest

Friday:

Aerobic Activity ____________________

Weight Training Workout Program ____________________

Weight Training Workout Routine ____________________

Or Rest

Saturday:

Aerobic Activity ____________________

Weight Training Workout Program ____________________

Weight Training Workout Routine ____________________

Or Rest

Sunday:

Aerobic Activity ____________________

Weight Training Workout Program ____________________

Weight Training Workout Routine ____________________

Or Rest

Workout Routine One	Reps	Weight
Leg Press		
Bench Press		
Calf Raises		
Pec Dec		
Crunches *		
Four-part Seated Row		
Reverse Crunches		NA
Shoulder Press		
Triceps Press-downs		
OR Triceps Extensions		
Biceps Curls		
Wrist Curls		
Reverse Wrist Curls		

* Note the weight only if you do crunches on an ab crunch machine. If you do crunches on a mat, leave the weight line blank.

Workout Routine Two	Reps	Weight
Leg Extentions		
Bench Press		
Leg Curls		
Pec Dec		
Calf Raises		
Four-part Seated Row		
Combo Crunches		NA
Shoulder Press		
Triceps Press-downs		
OR Triceps Extensions		
Biceps Curls		
Wrist Curls		
Reverse Wrist Curls		

My Workout Regimen

Week Five

Monday:

Aerobic Activity ____________________

Weight Training Workout Program ____________________

Weight Training Workout Routine ____________________

Or Rest

Tuesday:

Aerobic Activity ____________________

Weight Training Workout Program ____________________

Weight Training Workout Routine ____________________

Or Rest

Wednesday:

Aerobic Activity ____________________

Weight Training Workout Program ____________________

Weight Training Workout Routine ____________________

Or Rest

Thursday:

Aerobic Activity ____________________

Weight Training Workout Program ____________________

Weight Training Workout Routine ____________________

Or Rest

Friday:

Aerobic Activity ______________________________

Weight Training Workout Program ______________________________

Weight Training Workout Routine ______________________________

Or Rest

Saturday:

Aerobic Activity ______________________________

Weight Training Workout Program ______________________________

Weight Training Workout Routine ______________________________

Or Rest

Sunday:

Aerobic Activity ______________________________

Weight Training Workout Program ______________________________

Weight Training Workout Routine ______________________________

Or Rest

Workout Routine One	Reps	Weight
Leg Press		
Bench Press		
Calf Raises		
Pec Dec		
Crunches *		
Four-part Seated Row		
Reverse Crunches		NA
Shoulder Press		
Triceps Press-downs		
OR Triceps Extensions		
Biceps Curls		
Wrist Curls		
Reverse Wrist Curls		

* Note the weight only if you do crunches on an ab crunch machine. If you do crunches on a mat, leave the weight line blank.

Workout Routine Two	Reps	Weight
Leg Extentions		
Bench Press		
Leg Curls		
Pec Dec		
Calf Raises		
Four-part Seated Row		
Combo Crunches		NA
Shoulder Press		
Triceps Press-downs		
OR Triceps Extensions		
Biceps Curls		
Wrist Curls		
Reverse Wrist Curls		

Appendix Three

Exercise Instructions Quick Reference Charts

Aerobic Exercise Equipment *

Equipment	Instructions
Treadmill	Walk, jog or run. Vary elevation and speed.
Stationary Bike	Adjust the seat height. Vary resistance and speed.
Elliptical Stepper	Use vertical handlebars to increase intensity.
Stepper	Use entire foot or balls of feet. Vary resistance and speed.
Rowing Machine	Keep elbows close to sides. Avoid locking out elbows.

* Note: Consult Chapter Eight for complete discussion and important information about proper use.

Weight Training Exercises: Upper Body *

Muscle	Exercise	Movement
Chest	Vertical Bench Press	Push bar away until there's a slight bend in elbows. Allow bar to come back, controlling the weight.
Chest	Vertical Fly	Squeeze pads together. Stop before they touch. Return to starting position, controlling the weight.
Back	Seated Row	Keep arms extended and sit back Pull row handle toward abdomen Extend arms, controlling the weight. Lean in to starting position.
Shoulders	Shoulder Press	Press bar upward until just before lockout. Allow bar to come back down, controlling the weight.
Arms	Triceps Press-downs	Push bar down toward thighs by extending arms. Return to starting position, controlling the weight.
Arms	Triceps Extensions	Pull bar down toward tights by extending arms. Return to starting position, controlling the weight.
Arms	Biceps Curls	Curl bar up. Return to starting position (slight bend in elbows).
Arms	Wrist Curls	Flex (bend) wrists. Return to starting position.
Arms	Reverse Wrist Curls	Reverse curl wrists as arms bend at elbow. Uncurl wrists as arms straighten.

* Note: Consult Chapter Eleven for complete descriptions, illustrations and important notes about proper form.

Weight Training Exercises: Lower Body *

Muscle	Exercise	Movement
Legs	Leg Extensions	Extend legs to the point just before knees lock out. Return to starting position, controlling the weight.
Legs	Leg Curls	Curl the bar down and back as far as machine allows. Control the weight as bar comes back up.
Legs	Leg Press	Push footplate by extending legs. Don't lock out. Control footplate as it comes down.
Legs	Calf Raises	With legs extended, push footplate away from you. Allow heels to go under footplate.
Legs	Inner-Outer Thigh Pulls	To work adductors, bring legs together. To work abductors, spread legs apart.

* Note: Consult Chapter Eleven for complete descriptions, illustrations and important notes about proper form.

Weight Training Exercises: Abs *

Muscle	Exercise	Movement
Abs	Crunches (Mat)	Lift chest off mat, but don't bend at waist. Return to starting position slowly.
Abs	Reverse Crunches (Mat)	Curl knees toward chest. Lower knees slowly, stopping before feet touch mat.
Abs	Combo Crunches (Mat)	Simultaneously do a crunch and reverse crunch. Return to starting position slowly.
Abs	Crunches (Machine)	Move chest toward thighs. Return to starting position, controlling the weight.
Abs	Vertical Knee Raises	Lift both knees toward chest. Slowly lower knees to starting position.

* Note: Consult Chapter Eleven for complete descriptions, illustrations and important notes about proper form.

Stretches *

Muscle	Movement
Lower Back	Lie on back. Bring one knee toward chest. Clasp hands around hamstrings or lower leg. Pull knee toward chest
Lower Back	Lie on back. Bring both knees toward chest. Put one hand around each leg below kneecap, or both arms around both legs below kneecaps. Pull knees toward chest.
Quads	Lie on left side. Extend left arm. Bend right leg. Grasp right ankle with right hand. Bring right heel to buttocks. Keep legs parallel. Repeat on right side.
Quads	Stand straight. Place object on floor behind you. Bend right knee. Place toes on object. Keep legs parallel. Repeat with left leg.
Quads	Stand straight. Bend right leg. Grasp ankle with right hand. Bring heel close to buttocks. Keep legs parallel. Repeat with left leg.
Hams	Sit on mat with legs extended and together. Point toes toward ceiling. Bend from waist. Grasp any part of your legs that you can reach.
Hams	Place an object on floor in front of you. Keeping left leg straight, lift it and place heel on object. Repeat with right leg.
Calves	Stand six inches away from wall. Place hands on wall. Move one foot back as far as you can while keeping heel on floor. Repeat with other leg.
Calves	Stand a foot away from wall. Place hands on wall. Keep one leg straight. Place heel of other foot on floor as close to wall as possible. Repeat with other leg.

Stretches continued *

Muscle	Movement
Inner Thighs	Sit with back against wall. Bend both legs. Bring soles of feet together. Grasp ankles. Pull feet as close to body as possible.
Outer Thighs, Sides and Lower Back	Sit on mat with left leg extended. Bend right leg. Place right foot on floor outside of left knee so foot touches knee. Put right hand on floor in line with right hip. Put left elbow against outside of right leg at bend of knee. Rotate upper body and head to right. Gently push right leg to left with left elbow. Repeat on other side.
Shoulders, Upper Back and Triceps	Stand straight. Extend one arm across body under chin. Place palm of other hand on elbow of extended arm. Repeat with other arm.
Shoulders and Chest	Stand straight with feet shoulder width apart. Extend arms straight down behind you. Clasp hands.
Forearms	Stand straight. Extend arms in front of you. Rotate hands so palms face up. Rotate hands so backs face each other and thumbs point down. Bend right wrist so fingers point down and palm faces you. Place left hand across back of right hand. Gently pull right hand toward you. Bend right wrist so fingers point down and palm faces away from you. Place left hand across fingers of right hand. Gently pull right hand toward you. Repeat lines three through ten with left hand.
Upper Back and Sides	Stand straight with feet shoulder width apart. Raise arms above head. Grasp right wrist with left hand. Bend elbow slightly. Bend over to left while gently pulling right arm to left. Repeat on left side.
	Stretches continued on next page.

Stretches continued *

Muscle	Movement
Sides	Stand with feet shoulder width apart. Keep arms at sides. Bend from waist to the right. Repeat on other side.

* Note: Consult Chapter Fourteen for complete descriptions, illustrations and important notes about proper form.

Glossary

Aerobic exercise - Physical activity that is continuous, as opposed to stop and go (e.g., jogging, walking, cross-country skiing, non-competitive cycling and swimming). The body uses oxygen as its primary source of energy for these activities

Anaerobic exercise - Physical activity that is non-continuous and uses glucose, not oxygen, as the primary source of energy (e.g., weight training, competitive sports).

Antioxidants - Found in certain foods. Antioxidants destroy free radicals in the body, which damage DNA.

Atrophy - The state at which muscles waste away or weaken from lack of use.

Awesome Foursome, The - The essential components of optimal health and total fitness: sensible eating lifestyle, cardiovascular endurance training, muscle strength and endurance training, static stretching for flexibility.

Calorie - A unit of measurement for the energy released when the body breaks down the chemical bonds of food.

Carbohydrates, complex - Starchy foods that come mainly from plants and are healthful because they contain nutrients (vitamins and minerals) and fiber, and provide energy. Complex carbs are found in whole grain (wheat, oats, rye) breads and cereals, pasta, corn, fruits and vegetables, beans, peas and potatoes.

Carbohydrates, simple - Carbohydrates with simple structures that can easily be broken down into glucose. Simple carbohydrates are commonly referred to as sweets or sugars. Simple carbs are found naturally in fruits (fructose) and milk (lactose). Refined sugars are found in sweet desserts, chocolate, jams and jellies.

Cardiovascular (C/V) - endurance training - Regular aerobic exercise to increase the efficiency of your cardiovascular system, enabling you to engage in physical activity for longer periods of time without fatiguing. C/V endurance training also wards off certain medical conditions, and enhances your brain functioning.

Cartilage - Connective tissue that covers the ends of bones at the joints. It serves as a cushion, or shock absorber, to prevent bone on bone friction.

Cool-down - The period of activity that follows your workout. At the end of your cardio workout, gradually reduce the intensity and speed of your aerobic exercise for five minutes to cool down. After your weight-training workout, do your static stretching routine to cool down.

Definition - The contours or outline of muscles (i.e., the two parts of the biceps muscles are clearly defined).

Extensor muscles - Muscles that straighten limbs (e.g., quads, triceps).

Fat - Found in foods coming from animals, and in oils and butter.

Fiber - Consuming foods high in fiber (whole grains, fruits and vegetables) can lower blood pressure, reduce susceptibility to digestive problems, and diminish the risk of heart disease and diabetes. Another plus: foods high in fiber fill you up and reduce the urge to snack and overeat.

Flexibility - The ability to move freely and smoothly through full ranges of motion without pain or discomfort.

Flexor muscles - Muscles that bend limbs (e.g., hams, biceps)

Glucose - A simple sugar produced when the body breaks down carbohydrates. The glucose is then stored in your muscles so that it is immediately available for energy when needed. Glucose is also the brain's primary fuel. But the brain doesn't store glucose; it must be constantly available for optimal brain function.

High-density lipoprotein cholesterol (HDL) - The "good cholesterol." It can remove cholesterol from the blood and lower the risk of cardiovascular disease and stroke.

Hypertension - High blood pressure.

Interchangeable Aerobic Training (IAT) - Alternately changing the two intensity variables (speed and resistance/elevation) on aerobic exercise equipment without the use of a pre-set program.

Joint - Where two bones meet and movement takes place (e.g., elbow, knee, hip, shoulder).

Ligaments - Hold two bones together at joints.

Local muscular endurance - The length of time a muscle can keep contracting and causing movement before it succumbs to fatigue.

Locking out - Fully extending your arms or legs until you cannot go any further. You should never lock out a joint when weight training because it can damage cartilage, muscles, tendons and bones. Always stop when joints are slightly bent.

Low-density lipoprotein cholesterol (LDL) - The "bad" cholesterol. It increases the risk of cardiovascular disease and stroke.

Maximum heart rate (MHR) - 220 minus your age is your MHR. The fastest a human heart can beat is 220 times a minute, but we lose about one beat a minute for every year of life.

Momentary failure - When you lift weights you're inducing the momentary failure of muscles. When a muscle reaches momentary failure, you experience a sensation often referred to as "the burn." The burn is a reaction to the microscopic tearing of muscle fibers. The body repairs the microscopic muscle tears caused by momentary failure during your rest period. The repair process increases the size and strength of muscles in small increments.

Muscle strength and endurance training - Weight training to increase strength and improve local muscular endurance. Muscle strength and endurance training will not only enhance your performance in sports and other physical activities, but it will also make your daily activities easier and reduce your risk of injury.

Negative repetition (rep) - The second movement of any weight-training exercise.

Neutral position - The tops of your hands and the tops of your forearms make a straight line (no bend in your wrists).

Nutrients - Carbohydrates, fats, proteins, vitamins, minerals and water. They provide nourishment for our bodies to maintain, improve and restore health.

Positive repetition (rep) - The first movement of any weight-training exercise.

Power - The speed at which you can lift, push or pull a heavy weight. It's a function of time.

Protein - Found in nuts, lean animal tissue, fish and beans. Protein is used by the body for energy only when carbohydrates and fat are not available.

Range of motion (ROM) - A measure of the distance a joint can move. In the context of weight training, a complete range of motion means keeping a muscle under tension throughout every repetition.

Recovery rate - The length of time it takes your heart to return to its resting rate after being in your target zone during a workout.

Repetition (Rep) - Every time you do the positive and negative movement of an exercise, you've completed one repetition.

Resting heart rate (RHR) - Your heart rate after you've been sitting for ten to twenty minutes. To obtain a more precise measure of your RHR, take your pulse for three mornings before you get out of bed; the average is your RHR.

Saturated fat - Commonly called the "bad" fat, saturated fat raises LDL ("bad" cholesterol) and has been linked to heart disease. Examples of saturated fat include meat and dairy products, such as cheese and butter.

Sensible eating lifestyle - A practical, common sense approach to healthful eating. A sensible eating lifestyle focuses on health, not weight.

Set - A specific number of repetitions.

Sprain - Occurs when ligaments are overstretched or torn. Movement becomes impaired or painful.

Static stretching - Elongating muscles slowly, and holding the position for fifteen to twenty seconds. Static stretching will enhance your flexibility and help you avoid injury from physical activity as well as everyday movements.

Strain - Occurs when tendons or muscles are overstretched or torn. Movement is impaired and painful. Strains are often referred to as pulled muscles.

Strength - Determines how much weight you can lift, push or pull. Strength is based on the amount of force muscles can produce or how forcefully they can contract and cause movement against resistance.

Stretched Out Workout Week (SOWW) - Gives you nine days to fit in three total body (weight training) workouts and three or four cardio workouts. You can customize your workout schedule to accommodate changes in your daily, weekly or monthly routines.

Target zone (TZ) - 50% to 85% of your maximum heart rate. To increase your cardiovascular endurance, you must get your heart rate into your target zone and keep it there for twenty minutes three to four times a week.

Tendon - Connects muscles to bones.

Tone - The degree of firmness and tension in muscles.

Unsaturated fats - This type of fat has health benefits, such as lowering your LDL cholesterol level (LDL is known as the "bad" cholesterol, while HDL is the "good" one). Unsaturated fats can be divided into two broad categories: (1) monounsaturated fats, which are found in such oils as olive, peanut and canola, and (2) polyunsaturated fats, which are found in such oils as corn, safflower and walnut.

Warm-up - The period of aerobic exercise that precedes your workout. Begin your cardiovascular workout with a five-minute warm-up period to get your heart beating a little faster. During the warm-up, gradually increase the intensity of your activity incrementally. Engage in aerobic exercise for five to ten minutes before your weight training workout to warm up your muscles.

Yo-yo dieting - Chronic dieting, or cycling on and off diets. Yo-yo dieting fails to keep weight off and can even lead to additional weight gain in the long run.

Index

A

C

D

E

F

G

H

I

J

L